Reality

Acceptance

For Happier and Healthier Lives

Brian Kirwan

For my wife, who allowed me to accept all realities.

Table of Contents

Reality Acceptance Introduction

Are you living your happiest and healthiest life? Before you answer that question, I want you to think about where your answer comes from. Is your answer based on what you think is true or the reality of your happiness and health? Most of us will answer the question based on what we think others want to hear or what we want to be true. "Of course, I'm happy! Why? What have you heard?" The actual answer, most times, is, "I don't know." Unless you are living your life having accepted the reality of your health, knowledge, thinking, and behavior, the answer to this question will always be, "I don't know." This book is your guide to change "I don't know" to "I'm working on it."

You can only be your happiest and healthiest self if you understand and accept the reality of what being happy and healthy mean. Understanding what is real and accepting that reality are the first steps to solving any problems with your life. If you are miserable, stressed, anxious, angry, or dealing with other health problems, you can remove these barriers to your happiness and health by accepting the reality of them. Accepting the reality of your problems is only the beginning of changing your life for the better.

Reality Acceptance has changed my life. I am happier and healthier than I have ever been. I lived many miserable years when I was younger because I did not accept the reality of my life. My anxiety, anger, depression, loneliness, sensory issues, being overweight, and ignoring or denying issues made my reality denial worse. Our beliefs and opinions about ourselves and others are barriers to accepting reality and living our best life. We also fear change, but we forget we control how our lives change. No changes will happen without your consent or your understanding of the possibilities of the changes.

We all ignore, deny, or hide from realities we do not want to accept. Accepting that we need to lose weight is not enough if we do not accept our need to exercise or stop eating fast food. We justify our weight by telling ourselves we do not have the time, it is too expensive, or it is not important. None of these are true. We make choices in our lives based on these misunderstandings of reality. Reality Acceptance will help you realize these beliefs keep you from your best life.

Accepting reality is about understanding reality. If you lost your way in an unfamiliar area, you have experienced the difficulty of understanding unfamiliar realities. Roads, people, and buildings surround you, but you have little understanding of how they relate to you. You must become familiar with the realities of the area before you can understand them and find where you need to go. Your being lost is a problem you need to solve. Accepting the reality of the area is the first step to solving it.

The concept of Reality Acceptance seems simple. If we did not accept the reality of our lives, how would we get through our day? Getting through your life is not what this book is about. I want you to get through your life in the happiest and healthiest way you can. To do this, you need to accept the reality of your life. This means accepting your beliefs, biases, and hopes are not part of reality. They are your perceptions of reality. Understanding reality is tough because it represents everything. I will not explain everything in this book. I will explain how best to understand reality so you can solve any problem for yourself.

My goal in this book is to allow you to help yourself with the same steps that helped me. This is a self-help book, but it is also a problem-solving book. I do not want you to solve a few problems in your life. I want you to solve all the problems in your life. Once you have done that, I want you to help others solve problems in their lives. As with all self-help books, this book can only help you if you will help yourself. I have read many self-help books in creating this one. They accept the reality of the problem they are helping you solve, but none of them accept all of reality so you can solve all your problems.

Not all reality is easy to accept. Accepting the reality that you made yourself miserable may make you want to ignore or reject this knowledge. You may sink into the regrets of lost time in your life. This is not my goal in this book. If you have unrealistic beliefs about yourself or the world, they are preventing your progress in life. If you are unwilling to change those beliefs, this book will not help you. There are no magic pills in this book or in reality. Reading this book will get you started understanding the reality of your problems so you can solve them for yourself.

I have constructed the information in this book to teach you concrete steps for accepting reality. There are six parts I will focus on. Each part progresses from a personal examination of reality to a more social and inclusive view. **Part 1** will explain the basics of the concept of Reality Acceptance. **Part 2** includes chapters about **Health**. The most important reality to accept is your health. This includes your physical and mental health. **Part 3** includes chapters about

Knowledge. Science is the best tool humans have developed for understanding reality. **Part 4** includes chapters on **Thinking**. How you think about the world and what you believe will affect your ability to accept reality and solve problems. **Part 5** includes chapters on **Behavior**. Accepting other people, even if they think or act differently from you, is a large part of accepting reality. How you behave toward them will change how they behave toward you.

Part 6 and the last section includes chapters I call **Reality Accepted**. It concerns issues you will deal with once you have accepted the major realities in your life. How much reality is too much? Is all reality relevant to you? Can use Reality Acceptance to handle any problem? You will hopefully be able to answer these questions for yourself by the end of the book. Accepting the reality of an ever-changing world requires constant updates to the reality you accept. Once you understand what is real, you must deal with people who do not accept reality for themselves. My hope is you can help guide others through accepting reality by the end of this book. Enough with the introductions. Let us begin!

My Personal Reality Acceptance Journey

I always understood something was off in my life. I looked and acted similar to other people, but there was something not right. This confusing haze lasted about 48 years of my life. Now I have specificity for my confusing life. I discovered I have autism. Some people call it high-functioning autism, and some people dislike that term. I realized my view of the world was different because I perceived reality differently. Most people can ignore the world around them. Reality is not something I can escape or ignore easily. I have a heightened sense of reality compared to most people. This has made me an expert at accepting reality for what it is and dealing with it.

I am fascinated by science as a way of understanding reality. When I was younger, science offered a logical understanding of people and the world around me. It did not stop bullies from picking on me, but it offered me an understanding of their behavior. They ridicule others before they get ridiculed. I knew psychologically why they did this, but they were physically larger than me. I knew my scientific studies of people would not help me in a fight. Knowing they would pay the price for their simplistic views as adults did not protect me against their fists when I was young. The unpleasant behavior of these bullies seemed illogical because it was.

My journey toward reality acceptance began when I realized I was an atheist. It started with just not believing in God, but progressed until I realized I did not believe in any supernatural beings or religion as a concept. I knew all the cool supernatural beings like vampires, dragons, and wizards were not real, so why would I believe in uninteresting supernatural beings? The whole concept of worshiping God seemed negative. He seemed like a being who did not care about people until they needed smiting. The image of Jesus on the cross seemed out of a horror film, and I did not like horror films.

Eventually, I went from being angry at believers to feeling sorry for them. They were so focused on supernatural things that they did not notice the wonder of nature and reality around them. They would rather look at a religious building or statue than at the enormous variety of nature's wonders, such as trees, plants, and animals. A building constructed 100 years ago cannot compare to nature that developed over billions of years. Their beliefs were keeping them from experiencing realities that could improve their lives. They should question their beliefs because they are preventing them from being happy and healthy.

I am a caring atheist. I care about other people, but I do not concern myself with their beliefs unless those beliefs keep them from caring about others. All the major conflicts in the world have been from differing beliefs. People claim wars are for economic issues, land ownership, and resources, but the real catalyst for their actions are their beliefs. People hide their beliefs if they think those around them do not believe the same as they do. The people who believe hideous things are not hideous, their beliefs are.

From the time humans have interacted, their beliefs have separated them from other humans. I definitely separated myself from other people because of my beliefs. If I disagreed with other people's beliefs, I knew why their beliefs were wrong. I did not have the same awareness of my own beliefs. My beliefs were guesses about the world I was living my life by. I thought I was using my experiences, problem-solving skills, and knowledge, but I was using my beliefs to guess my way through each day.

In high school, my parents went through a bankruptcy because of a failed business. This negative event forced me to accept realities I had not confronted in the past. I had to put myself through college, drive whatever car my parents did not need, and live a stripped-down life to which I was unaccustomed. The college I went to did not have a football team or frats, but it had students who knew the importance of the education they were getting. After five years, I graduated with a four-year degree in English Composition. My degree seemed useless, but it has served me well in my life.

I accepted reality in my writing long before I accepted reality in my life. We must live life in chronological order while I could write in a random order as thoughts occurred to me and organize them later. My mind works randomly. I could work through problems by writing about them much easier than I could work on them at other times in my life. As time went on, I could transfer my skills in writing to the rest of my life. Writing taught me to organize my thoughts into categories. Once organized, I could express them to others more clearly.

I have written my observations about the world most of my life. Eventually, I focused my thoughts into a general acceptance of reality. As I collected similar thoughts into distinct categories, four of them emerged: **Health**, **Science**, **Thinking**, and **Other People Exist**. I have written about science, health, and thinking throughout most of my life. When I wrote about my interactions with other people, it developed into **Other People Exist**. If you did not agree with other people about science, health, or thinking, you could agree that other people exist. The categories eventually became **Health**, **Knowledge**, **Thinking**, and **Behavior**. You must accept the reality of your health, knowledge, thinking, and behavior to accept reality completely.

As a young adult, I accepted the reality of my health. I noticed a correlation between eating sugar and getting acne, so I stopped eating sugar. The acne went away. I also stretched and exercised regularly. Periodically, I stopped exercising, but I always stretched. To this day, I am still more flexible than most of the people I know, regardless of their age. Several years ago, I started eating a vegan diet. I allow myself to cheat when I am on vacation. Despite exercising, I noticed a dip in my health after a vacation. I have never broken a bone, have no lingering aches or pains, and I walk up and down stairs rather than ride an elevator. On the other side, I am losing my hearing in one ear, I still struggle with my posture, and I do not get enough sleep most of the time. I am not as healthy as I could be. There is always room for improvement and more reality to accept.

I am hoping to use what I have learned in my journey toward accepting reality to expand the concept of Reality Acceptance with the help of others. Only by accepting other perspectives on reality can Reality Acceptance grow as a concept. My goal is to allow the greatest number of people to enjoy happier and healthier lives and to make Reality Acceptance an accepted term by both scientific and non-scientific people alike. I am not claiming I am taking a scientific examination of reality, but I based the concepts on established science. I hope Reality Acceptance will continue to improve long after my journey ends.

Part 1
Reality Acceptance Explained

Chapter 1

What is Reality Acceptance?

Accept reality for what it is, not what you want it to be. People and groups who deny reality do so because reality is against them in their minds. Reality is not their friend. If you dislike how the world is, deny it is that way. If you do not agree with someone else, deny anything they say has validity. We all perceive reality differently and interpret what we perceive differently. To accept reality, you must become a reality detective. We do not perceive reality in simple to understand presentations. Our experiences, senses, and beliefs mask reality. We can only understand reality by gathering the perceptions of others and matching them with our own. Life will present you with many problems to solve in your life. Accepting reality will lead to better outcomes for these problems.

Examining reality is difficult. Most of us have spent a life with beliefs, biases, and a singular point of view about the world. Widening your focus to see the reality of any situation requires accepting a diverse group of perceptions. Reality Acceptance is a skill you must develop. I will help you accept reality, but I will not explain reality. If I claimed to explain reality, you would know I was lying. I will give you the skills to discern reality even when your senses, experiences, and beliefs tell you something different.

Accepting reality is about accepting limitations. If you do not see the limits of something, you are only missing the limits. Everything has limits. You must work with the limits to accomplish what you want in life. People see limits as barriers they must avoid, but they are just the parameters of reality. The possibilities between the limits are much more abundant than people believe. Accomplishing goals within these limits is possible if they are realistic. Working with limitations builds your creativity and problem-solving skills.

An important part of accepting reality is a concept I call Other People Exist. You cannot accept reality without acknowledging the feelings and experiences of other people. Our individual experiences only allow us a limited view of reality. Even the other people you see regularly only widen your view slightly. If you separate yourself from other people, you are separating yourself from reality. Understanding reality is gathering a diverse number of experiences directly or through other people. Connecting to other people helps us understand them and ourselves better.

I accept the reality of the world and am a happier person because of it. I see other people whose beliefs, experiences, and biases lead to a miserable life. Nothing about reality is miserable, but their view of it only allows them to see negativity in the world. The more you examine reality, the more you will see how few things are inherently negative. Your misery is completely in your head and has nothing to do with reality. Happiness is a choice we must learn to accept. If no one taught you to accept reality, you never will.

Reality Acceptance Categories Explained

Accepting all of reality is my goal in life, but I know it is unattainable. To accept all of reality would take the rest of my life and I would never fully understand all of it. Luckily, you and I only have to accept the reality of the world we deal with directly. There are some complex realities we will never understand, but they are unnecessary to achieving happiness and health. Accepting what we can know and what we cannot is part of accepting reality.

I arranged the parts of this book from simple personal realities to more complex realities involving other people. You must deal with your **Health** before you can accept the **Knowledge** science can teach us. You can use this knowledge to examine your **Thinking**. Accepting the reality of how you think leads to accepting the reality of your **Behavior** toward other people who have distinct ways of thinking. I made this journey toward Reality Acceptance without the benefit of the book. The lessons of accepting reality came in a random order. I took those random lessons and ordered them so you can accept reality for yourself.

The first part of accepting reality is accepting the reality of your **Health**. Ill health will hamper your perception of reality. As your health improves, you will be happier, and your view of life will improve. Most people would benefit by examining their health more closely. You can only work on health problems you accept as real. You can start with your physical body. Are you dramatically over or under weight? Do you have frequent illnesses or health problems? Do you eat nutritious food and exercise? The answers to these questions will tell you the state of your physical health. Next, start thinking about your mental health. Are you a content person? Do you have anxiety, depression, anger, confusion, or other issues preventing you from being happy? The answers to these questions will tell you the state of your mental health. The reality of your health requires working on both your physical and mental health to improve your overall health.

Knowledge can help you improve your physical and mental health as long as you accept the reality science can teach. Science examines reality without bias, opinions, or inconsistencies. Science allows everyone to gain knowledge about the world without having to conduct experiments themselves. Examining established science will allow you to understand reality. All scientific information gets updated, re-examined, and questioned by other scientists. Science is constantly developing and growing. Our understanding of reality grows with it. Science examines what we cannot perceive with our senses alone. The knowledge learned from science can help you understand and accept reality.

Your **Thinking** about the world will improve your perception and knowledge of reality. Knowing why you think as you do is much more important than expressing simple but clear thoughts about what you believe. Filling your head with the thoughts of others will only result in thinking like they do. If they think negatively, you will have negative thoughts. Reality is neither positive nor negative, it is a mix of both. Focusing on the positive aspects of life will give you a positive outlook on life. As your thinking becomes more positive, it will cause your behavior to improve. This will improve your relationships with other people and the world.

When you accept the existence of other people, your **Behavior** toward them will affect them as much as it does you. Your positive interactions with other people will improve until you and the other people are happier and healthier. You will notice others who are not happy or healthy because they are not accepting the reality of their life. If you know them, you can try slowly to get them to accept more realities to improve their lives. Some will resist or deny reality, but others will accept the realities in their lives. Through your journey of Reality Acceptance, you will have learned the skills of living a happy and healthy life so you can spread reality acceptance to others.

The Benefits of Reality Acceptance

The top benefits of **Reality Acceptance** are living a happier and healthier life. Only by accepting reality can you improve your life for the better. You can accept the reality of your life, whether it is positive or negative. Many people have a harder time accepting the positive aspects of reality than the negative. People expect reality to be negative, but most of it is not. Ignoring or denying reality will only allow the negative aspects of life to continue or get worse. By accepting reality, you can deal with problems while they are small. The more reality you accept, the better your life will become.

You will improve your happiness.

The key to improving your happiness is knowing what makes you happy. If you are not a content person, you are not aware of what makes you happy. What you think makes you happy may not make you happy. Many people blame others when they are not happy. If they had enough money, were more attractive, had more control over their lives, or were smarter, they would be happy. The only person who can make you happy is you.

You will improve your health.

Your health does not change based on random factors. The two most crucial factors of physical health are nutrition and exercise. They are not the only factors involved in health, however. Your mental health is just as important as your physical health. Accepting the reality of your health is accepting the mental and physical factors that improve your health and avoiding factors that degrade your health.

You will value your limited time.

Valuing your time and the time of others will vastly improve your life. Accepting the limitation of time allows you to prioritize your time by what is actually important. Wasting time on ignoring or denying reality is wasting your limited time.

You will slow your life down.

We hurry through life without looking at the wonders of the world. Some of us are speeding our way on the highway and others are running from line to line so we can wait impatiently for our life to resume. We think we are saving time speeding through life, but we never live the life we are speeding toward. Another benefit of slowing down is saving money on speeding tickets.

You will have less stress.

Nothing in life is inherently stressful. Accepting stress into your life is the same as accepting happiness. You can perceive any situation in a positive or negative way. Some situations come with a certain amount of pressure, but the only things you need to focus on are the problems that need solutions. If you focus too much on the pressure you are feeling, you will exhaust yourself before you can solve any problems.

You will have less depression.

An extreme amount of negative thinking can cause depression. Your negative thinking feeds on negative events in your life, causing you to think even more negatively. The reality of the world is more pleasant than most people perceive. Seeing negative aspects of the world requires ignoring or denying most of reality. If you feel alone, it is because you are choosing to not connect with other people.

You will have fewer illnesses.

Most illnesses emanate from habits that begin in childhood. People focus on the germs, diseases, and injuries that cause an illness without looking at the reality of their health. The genuine cause of most illnesses is a lack of nutrition or exercise, stress, depression, anxiety, anger, and other unhealthy activities. Accepting only the direct cause of your illness discounts the reality that led to it.

You will have less anxiety.

I was a shy child with much anxiety. If I could have accepted the reality of my world, I could have accepted the things I was anxious about and dealt with them before they became worse. Accepting your anxiety is key to solving the problems in your life that cause the anxiety.

Less hatred will exist in the world.

One of my hopes for this book is to remove the word "hate" from the vocabulary of those who read it and those who care about them. Hate is a word that is only negative. People hate Mondays because it is usually the day people go back to work after the weekend. Mondays are problem days for them, but the word "hate" is too strong. Especially when you hate another person, you are setting yourself up for problems when dealing with that person. When you accept reality, you will no longer find things to hate in the world. Hate will become a useless word in your life, and you will notice only hateful and miserable people using it.

You will improve your self-esteem.

Low self-esteem may stem from others telling you how worthless you are, but staying around those people is completely up to you. If you convinced yourself you are worthless by listening to negative people, start listening to positive people who can convince you of your worth. Everyone who is reading this can be happy and healthy. Pursuing things that make you happy and healthy will improve your self-esteem.

You will improve the quality of your life.

Accepting reality allows you to deal with problems before they become negative aspects of your life. The more you accept, the more you will notice the interesting parts of life. You will become interested in life and other people. Your interest in other people will then improve their lives.

Your curiosity will continue regardless of your age.

If we are not curious about the world, we are not curious about life. A lack of curiosity can lead to boredom, ignorance, or depression. Reality is the most diverse and exciting experience consciousness provides us. Curiosity builds enthusiasm for life.

You will learn to recognize the help available to you.

We have support systems around us we do not recognize. We assume no one wants to help us. This leads to not asking or looking for help. We are far more willing to help one another than we believe. If we do not get help from others, we have not asked for it.

You will become a better friend.

Friendships are important for your mental health. Genuine friends are people who care about each other in the best and worst of times. They accept one another without judgment. Arguing with a friend does not end the relationship. You can lie to your boss, but lying to your friend could end the friendship. Learning to be more accepting of yourself and others will allow you to be a better friend.

You will remove irrelevant information from your life.

This book is not about accepting all known information about the world and the creatures who inhabit it. Most information is neither interesting nor relevant to your life. We all have a limited amount of time in our lives, so valuing time means limiting irrelevant information. If the information does not affect your health or your happiness, you are okay not knowing it.

You will improve your problem-solving skills.

Solving problems is the most important thing you can learn in life. Being able to translate all your life-experience into a new context is a skill that will serve you well. Accepting the reality of your past and present experiences will develop this skill. We do not solve most problems in isolation. The more experience you have solving problems, the more help you can be to others.

You will be more attractive to other people.

Happy and healthy people are the most attractive people. You attract people to you because you are pleasant to be around. Beauty is only skin deep, and it has nothing to do with how appealing you are as a person. A sunset is beautiful, but people are attractive to you because they make you happy. Happiness is appealing.

Reality Acceptance Basics

Accepting reality begins with the basics of reality. The following is a starter kit for accepting reality. They are basic steps you can take to begin your journey into **Reality Acceptance**. If you do one of these a day, you will quickly improve your happiness and health.

- Remove negative words from your vocabulary.
- Instead of saying what should be, accept what is and change it.
- If you follow the news, stop. It is not good for your health.
- Avoid negative people.
- Start accepting the positive aspects of reality and your life.
- Stop lying to yourself.
- Stop lying to others.
- Value your own time.
- Value the time of others.
- Accept the reality of your health.
- Accept ambiguity. It will be okay even without all the answers.
- Notice what makes you happy.
- Learn how you can improve your health.
- Notice when and why you get stressed.

- Avoid unhealthy behaviors.

- Notice when and why you get angry, depressed, or anxious.

- Do not express opinions about things you do not understand.

- Avoid extreme points of view and thinking.

- Accept the unknown.

- Avoid advertisements.

- Learn something new every day.

- Be curious about other people and the world.

- Notice the positive behavior around you.

Reality Accepting Exercise:

At the end of each chapter, I will have an exercise that points out how the ideas from the chapter can help you accept the reality I describe. This first exercise is to try out some of the Reality Acceptance Basics in your daily life.

Chapter 2
Reality Acceptance in the Real World

Valuing Time

Valuing time is an important concept in this book and in life.
We can work together in society if we consider our own time
and that of others. We all have a limited time on earth.
Valuing time means making the most of your limited time.
When you ignore or deny reality, you are not valuing time.
The goal of valuing time is being happy and healthy for the
greatest percentage of your life.

When I was a kid, I saw other kids wasting their time
bullying other kids, worrying about who liked them, or seeing
what they could get away with. Far from valuing their time,
they were wasting their childhoods. The most valuable activity
was playing with other kids and developing friendships, but
they wanted to rush their way into adulthood. Becoming an
adult happens too quickly on a regular time scale. Enjoying
being a kid allows you to appreciate these carefree times when
you are older.

You will neglect most aspects of your life if you only
focus on a few. Spending more time on one aspect will leave
less time for others. Focusing only on your career will neglect
your personal life, relationships, and your health. You must
distribute your time evenly and efficiently, or you will find
yourself unfulfilled in your life. Widen your focus in life and
you will discern what values your time. Ignoring realities you
find unimportant will lead to negative consequences for
realities you find important.

Sitting and doing nothing does not automatically lead to boredom. Spending time alone is valuable for you and the people in your life. Having your own thoughts and opinions is important for valuing yourself. If all of your thoughts and opinions come from others, you are acting as a mouthpiece for them. Valuing yourself as an individual is as important as valuing the time you spend with others. Our boredom is a symptom of being boring people. One regret people have when looking back on their lives is not living true to themselves. Be the person who brings value to others.

Planning how you spend your life is critical to valuing time. If you do not plan for the future, your time will become less valuable. Planning allows you to optimize your time. When planning for the future, keep in mind why you are planning. If you are planning to spend more time at work to make more money, you will regret that decision at the end of your life. Time with your family and friends will value your time more. You must balance your plans for the future, learn from the past, and live in the present.

Arbitrary time restraints can limit your ability to value time. Most arbitrary time restraints are self-imposed. If you say you do not have time to do things that value your time, that is an arbitrary time restraint. Part of valuing your time is arranging your time to prioritize what is valuable to you and those you care about. People making unrealistic demands upon their time will make unrealistic plans. Saying you do not have time to do something is focusing on the time restraint instead of what you are doing with your time. Prioritizing your time involves when, how, and what you do with your time. Dealing with arbitrary time restraints is a waste of time.

The top goal of valuing time is being content in your life. Being content has more to do with your choices than the reality you cannot change. Knowing what makes you happy is not always clear. If you do not know what makes you happy, you will not be content. Happiness differs from pleasure. Pleasure is brief, but happiness can grow throughout your lifetime. Planning to be happy and content is just as important as any other plan you will do. Valuing your time will increase how content you are.

An additional benefit of valuing time is better health. Balancing your time between exercise and good nutrition is just as important as valuing your happiness. Happiness will lead to better health, and good health will lead to greater happiness. Making time to eat right and exercise is a matter of starting slow and building. If you exercise too much when you start, you risk injuring yourself or stopping exercise all together because you are in pain. Nutrition can also take time to work into your routine. The end goal of developing healthy habits slowly is to make the habits part of your daily routine.

When unhealthy practices tempt you, having a plan is important. Your temptations will decrease as healthy practices become your routine, but they will never go away completely. If you are dealing with emotional problems, the temptations will increase. Reminding yourself of the healthy and unhealthy feelings will help. Sometimes we need to reward our positive behavior, and other times we need barriers to our negative behavior. Valuing your health will increase your happiness and extend your life.

Throughout my driving career on the freeways of California, I accumulated many speeding tickets. They were never over one or two a year, but they definitely showed that I was rushing my way through life. Every trip on the freeway was a race against time. Other drivers hit me from behind in two major accidents, one of which totaled my car. This was a wake-up call to me. With my next car, I learned I could improve my miles per gallon the slower I drove. Focusing on that took my focus away from speeding. Since that time, I have not had one speeding ticket.

Being in a hurry does not value your time. Life is a journey, so do not rush through it. We rush to an experience, during an experience, and away from an experience. We never experience the experience. Value the limited time you have on earth and the positive experiences you have in life. We can only live in the present. Our memories are in the past and we can speculate about the future, but life happens in the present. Many people have a habit of hurrying through their day. They feel they are late when they are not. The greatest gift we can give ourselves is slowing down and looking around.

Valuing time encompasses every activity in your life. At any point in your day, you can ask yourself, "Am I valuing my time right now?" Some things that value our time are music, reading, learning, relaxing, laughing, and exercising. They are all activities we can feel good doing because they are good for our physical and mental health. Valuing time is not about making the most of every moment, it is about valuing a high percentage of your lifetime. Valuing your own time includes valuing the time of others. Isolated people are not valuing their time.

You will have negative moments in your life, but how much those moments maintain or decrease your happiness is up to you. If you lose someone you care about, you can value those people in your memories. Focusing only on the loss is not valuing those people or your time. The only person who can say if you are valuing your time is you. You must accept the reality that time is finite. Valuing time is an important part of accepting reality.

Widen Your Focus

Focusing your attention on only one thing neglects everything else, including your happiness and health. Whether you only focus on politics, money, science, religion, health, food, or another singular aspect of life, other things in your life will suffer. Expand your focus and you will expand your mind. Rather than becoming an expert on one thing, learn as much as you can about many things. Other people exist beyond who you currently know. Get to know them as people, not stereotypes or cliches. Widening your focus will cause far fewer regrets at the end of your life.

Kids spend most of their time focusing on one thing at a time. This is not so much a choice as a limited ability to focus on multiple things at once. Kids have the excuse of being kids, but we should teach them to widen their focus as they grow up. Parents who focus their kids on a singular goal are doing them a disservice. Kids need to learn a variety of social skills to be happy in adult life. By only focusing on one or two non-social skills, the child's quality of life will decrease. Some parents unintentionally teach their kids to only focus on themselves. We call these kids brats. Hopefully, they grow up and deal with people outside their family and friends so they can widen their focus to other people. If they do not, we call these people self-centered.

Is widening my focus going to make me more successful? Being a well-rounded person will make you much more of an interesting and happy person, but it will not make you more successful unless you consider happiness being successful. Most people consider money to be the measure of success. If you want to be more successful financially or just more powerful, narrow your focus. People who have enormous amounts of money have it because they were born into money or they narrowed their focus so much that money was the only thing they focused on. They may have had divorces in their past, lost family and friends, lied to others, or suffered health problems, but they had money. You pay the price for wealth with your health, happiness, relationships, and everything you cannot buy with money.

In my angry atheist days, I would narrowly focus on religious groups I hated. If I found out someone was strongly religious, I would confront them about their religion or distance myself from them. I focused so narrowly on their religious views; I did not see them as people. Eventually, I did not prejudge them for what I thought were their views. Many religions narrowly focus only on religious issues and ignore issues outside this focus. I was doing the same with atheism. When I saw people as people and did not concern myself with their views on religion, I could relate to them as the wide variety of people they were.

Those who choose to narrow their focus in life will soon find themselves unable to widen their focus to the world at large. Widening your focus is a skill you must develop. If you never develop these skills, you will soon only see the narrow focus of the world you created. Everything else becomes invisible. Widening your focus means accepting the world around you and the people in it. The world around you is not going away, so you may as well embrace it and increase your awareness of other people. The more you pay attention to others, the more you will know them. Every negative view of other people will become more positive when you get to know them.

In high school, I saw many other classmates who were focusing all their attention on partying, drinking, and drugs. I escaped most of these things by being nerdy and shy. I remember one student who could remember everything he had ever learned. Most of the time, he did not have to study. He began coming to class stoned regularly. He was a military brat who recently spent time in Hawaii where he developed the habit. I never saw him beyond high school, but I imagine he lived a regular life with a regular job. Who knows how far he could have gone if he had not developed this habit? I always thought it was sad to see someone with extraordinary abilities choose to live an ordinary life.

Addictions are an extreme over-narrowing of your focus. When you only focus on one substance or one activity in your life, you can become addicted to it at the expense of the rest of your life. No substance or activity starts as an addiction. The more focus you give to one thing, the more your addiction can develop. We often need an intervention to break the narrow focus of the addiction. Just as you narrowed your focus to gain the addiction, you must widen your focus to break the addiction. We should avoid friends who share our addiction. We should accept friends and family members who can help you with your addiction. People who have been through your addiction can help you avoid making the same mistakes they did. Family and friends can also help you with moral support.

Moving forward without looking around you is ignoring life. When you narrowly focus on your career, making money, or anything that is not adding to your happiness or health, you are advancing one part of your life at the expense of the rest. Only looking forward allows you to hope for a future that may not happen. If you cannot be happy and healthy today, why do you think you will be happy and healthy tomorrow? Believing things will be better tomorrow is ignoring the reality of today. Until you are happy today, you cannot be happier tomorrow. Widening your focus will expand your view of the happiness already in your life.

Craving Simplicity in a Complex World

Most people dislike things that are complex. We crave simple things like sugar, salt, pleasure, and winning. Reality is nothing but complex systems interacting with other complex systems. In reality, nothing is simple if you scrutinize it long enough. People are only simplifying their view of reality when they attempt to simplify things in their life. Metaphors are examples of this simplification to explain complex subjects. When something becomes too complex, people ignore or deny the complexity. Because they do not understand the complex realities, they accept simpler explanations they can understand. Complex realities become unaccepted while we accept simple beliefs about reality. Their craving for simplicity overshadows their view of reality.

Complex realities do not make them unknowable. The only reality people need to understand is the reality they interact with. The average person need not understand the vastness of space or the interactions of microorganisms.

Understanding the reality of your health, relationships with others, and everyday problems only requires a basic grasp of reality. Depending on the amount of reality you accept, understanding reality at a basic level is possible. Although reality is complex, individuals need not understand every aspect.

I am not a fan of multiple-choice or "what if" questions. They often ask complex questions that simple answers do not answer sufficiently. I understand the importance of the concepts involved in most questions, but find the simplification of issues incompatible with my way of thinking. Making me choose between a few preset answers limited the essay worth of answers I could give to most questions. I crave more complex questions and answers in a world of simple questions and answers.

Facts do not matter as much as understanding general concepts. Individual facts, names, and numbers are useful when talking to someone about specific details of a subject, but they are unnecessary for basic levels of understanding. We need not speak a language with fluency to communicate with others. Some people like me cannot remember factual information well, but we can talk endlessly about any subject. We understand how the world works without memorizing the names and facts of what we are talking about. Reciting facts about something is not understanding that thing.

Simple solutions only work on simple problems. The more factors involved in a problem, the more complex a solution must be. When people propose simple solutions for complex problems, they ignore many factors. The simple solution may work briefly or with a limited amount of people, but a solution considering all factors will resolve problems for the most people. We must make compromises in dealing with complex problems. We cannot solve some problems to everyone's satisfaction. The goal in solving a complex problem is solving as high a percentage of the problem for the most people. Complex solutions are not as satisfying as simple solutions, but they are necessary for handling complex problems.

Sensible and well-thought-out strategies work better than simpleminded strategies. If you quickly create a strategy, it will be a simple strategy. A well-thought-out plan will always consider more factors than a simple one. You may not always have the luxury of time for a well-thought-out plan. Emergency situations require quick and simple solutions. A quick and simple strategy should be general enough to work in most emergency situations. Most situations in life are not emergencies.

Being late to somewhere is not an emergency. If you are speeding in and out of traffic, you have chosen a simple strategy for making quick and simple decisions. If you get into an accident, your unnecessary and highly preventable behavior will be at fault, not an actual emergency. Emergency situations can be stressful and harmful to your health. If you are purposely putting your brain into emergency mode without an emergency, you are stressing out your body for no reason. Save the stress of an emergency for an emergency.

Years ago, I found myself in charge of Adult and Youth Sports at the Recreation Center where I worked. The only problems I had were with Adult Sports. Even though it was a recreational league, some people took the games seriously. They argued with the calls of the umpires, injured themselves, and fought with other players. Their competitive thinking removed what I thought was the most important part of the game, having fun. Their singular focus on the competition of the game missed the point of forming relationships, getting exercise, and working together. They saw the world as win or lose and they did not like being losers. Winning is only important to those who see themselves as losers.

There are no exact opposites. Conservatives are not the opposite of Liberals, black is not the opposite of white, and there are no winners and losers in life. Competition has simplified our view of reality. Sports, politics, and economics have led us to believe we can reduce everything to simple yes or no answers. This all-or-nothing thinking ignores complex realities in favor of a simplified and unrealistic view of reality. Yes or no answers work for simple questions, but simple questions do not work for most of reality. Scientific test results are rarely 100% or 0%. Reality comprises so many factors that absolutes are rare if they exist at all.

Craving simplicity is not a problem as long as you accept the complexity of the world. We need not understand complexities to accept them. Complex problems involve many factors, including the people involved in a problem. Each person will have multiple factors to consider in finding a satisfactory solution for them. The more people involved, the more complex the solution needs to be. Simple solutions cannot solve complex problems any more than complex solutions are necessary for simple problems. Accepting a general reality will help you more than simple solutions that do not address all the factors involved in a problem.

Reality Accepting Exercise:

Think about where you are in your life right now. Are you valuing your time and the time of those in your life? Are you narrowly focused on your job, family, or even yourself? Think about the things you are not focusing on. What are you neglecting in the rest of your life? Think of ways to balance your time and widen your focus to your whole life.

Chapter 3

Reality Acceptance in a Reality Denying World

Accepting reality is easier now than it has ever been. I can state that regardless of when you read these words. We have been able to accept realities we did not know existed before. Human history has had many grim times concerning reality, but the world is accepting more reality every day. There are fewer wars, less poverty and starvation, and people are more educated. I am not saying people do not deny or ignore reality, but the more realities we accept, the better we can understand it. Despite how many people currently accept reality, many more do not.

The main reality denial remaining today concerns complex realities. In some people's minds, we explain the complexities of the universe through religion. Love, feelings of the heart, loyalty, pride, honor, and dreams are all concepts we only experience in our minds. People believe in them because they have positive associations with them, but they do not exist in a physical sense. We express these feelings by caring about and behaving kindly to others, but they are only real in that we can describe them. These mind experiences will not usually affect people negatively. If they lead to feelings of hatred, jealousy, anger, depression, or anxiety, then negative behaviors toward others will result. Believing these feelings are real and justified will lead to more negative behaviors.

Reality denying beliefs have shifted in recent years from worshiping supernatural beings to the worshiping of wealth. Much of this is a carryover from religious beliefs. Many religions have ornate churches, statues, temples, and the mansions of religious leaders who do not hide their worshiping of wealth. Most politicians, stars, and people who have an influence in the world are wealthy. By singularly focusing on the accumulation of wealth, they have ignored or denied other realities unless they affect their wealth.

Most people do not question the power of the wealthy because they are striving to become wealthy themselves. They look up to the wealthy as successful people who have achieved the dream they hold. Success is only measuring the accumulation of wealth, not the accumulation of life satisfaction. Having wealth without life satisfaction will lead to many regrets at the end of your life. In the current world, money needs to be a factor in your life, but it should not negatively affect your life-satisfaction. You are focusing too much on wealth if it does.

Many people feel accepting reality only means accepting the negative aspects of it. Bad days, angry people, and negative thoughts are regular parts of their perceptions. Your denial of it is a defense mechanism against the realities you would rather not confront. The positive aspects of reality far exceed the negative. If you are only focusing on the negative ones, you are ignoring most of reality. Accepting reality involves noticing the positive aspects of life. Our beliefs lead us to only see negative realities. When you accept reality, you will experience far less negativity in your life and in your thinking.

Accepting reality is possible with people who deny it, but it will not be easy. They are like other people; they simply deny realities others accept. Someone who is speeding in a school zone is not accepting the reality of that situation. He focuses on himself and does not accept the safety of the situation. You should not drag yourself into his denial by getting angry at him. If you know him, you might convince him to accept the reality of the situation. You will not get him to change his behavior if you do not. The best policy for reality denying strangers is to avoid them as much as possible. You will not get them to accept reality and they will not get you to deny it.

Accepting reality when raised in a family or group that denies many realities can be difficult. If your family is your only source for interpreting the world, you will accept the reality they present. Finding other sources, especially when you are young, is important to understanding true reality. You may need to conceal your thoughts if you depend on your family for support. As you grow older, you will know what realities they can accept. You must deal with their reality denial with compassion and understanding. They do not see themselves as denying reality. If their denial is harming you physically or mentally, you may need to get away from them to keep yourself safe.

When you are fully away from your reality denying family, you may eventually want to confront them about their reality denial. Just as you did not see their reality denial as positive, they will not see your reality acceptance as positive. You should not lie to them if they ask about your beliefs, nor should you speak negatively about their beliefs. Their reality denial has more to do with their beliefs and emotions than their ignorance of reality. Even if they were unkind to you as a child, it was because of the emotions they denied. You may never change their beliefs, but you can help them with their emotions.

Reality denial is more of a mental health problem than most people will admit. Treat your family as you would treat someone with a mental health issue, but do not be patronizing. Find simple truths you and your family members can agree on and slowly work to continue finding common understandings about reality. If their reality denial is not causing them immense physical or mental harm, you can let them know you care about them and you are there if they need you. The only help that may help them is therapy, which they will refuse.

The more a culture separates itself from other cultures, the more they are likely to be a cult. A cult is a culture that cuts itself off from other cultures. Many cultures do this, but we only consider them a cult if they cut themselves off to an extreme extent. The more you cut yourself off from others outside your culture, the more cult-like your life will be. You may not realize how isolated you are until you interact with other people outside your culture.

Children raised in cults are the most extreme version of how dangerous denying reality can be. If the beliefs of the cult are the only representations of reality they see, they will not know to question them. Most groups formed around beliefs are reality denying groups, but cults deny basic realities of the society they live in. They physically, mentally, and culturally separate themselves from the rest of society.

Secrets are a key component of cults to separate them from non-members. The leaders of cults keep secrets from their members, the members keep secrets from their family, and many cults keep secrets from the government. Most religions do not want you learning about another religion or non-religious teachings. A cult physically and mentally separates you from learning about non-cult teachings. Cults are extreme forms of groups formed around beliefs, but they point out the problem with these groups.

How can you avoid reality denial and reality deniers? As you accept reality, you will still need to interact with reality denial in various forms. Recognizing reality denial will allow you to avoid denying realities yourself. We should avoid people who are extreme reality deniers. When I denied reality in my past, I would try to teach other drivers a lesson by slowing them down on the freeway. I know now the freeway is not a proper place to give life lessons to my fellow drivers. It is best to avoid reality deniers as much as possible, especially if they are being unsafe.

Some groups who deny reality are so intolerable that more than avoiding the group is necessary. The group can harm you, loved ones, or total strangers using physical and/or mental torture. If you do not live in a free society, you may have few options available to you to help the situation. Even in a free society, being a minority or in another marginalized group can bring harm to you and your family. Finding an organization or group unaffiliated with the group denying reality may be necessary. The outside group can use the power of their organization to combat the harm done. An individual should never put themselves in danger by confronting a reality denying group alone. You can only help others if you are alive and well.

Reality Denial Exposed

My name is Brian, and I am a reality denier. I fully admit I have denied many realities in my life. I denied the realities of my sensory difficulties, emotional issues, speeding problems, and isolation from others. These are only a few of the realities I have denied in my life. I was not consciously aware of my denial, but they led to unhealthy behaviors that lowered my level of life satisfaction. I have been so unsatisfied with my life that I thought about suicide. My denial of reality caused these problems to arise.

Once you accept more realities, you will notice people denying realities everywhere. Where you find unhappy and unhealthy people, you will find reality denying people. Your happiness is completely up to you. Unhappy people can be in the same situation as a content people. Unhappy people will blame everyone else for their misery. Content people accept the reality of any situation without preconceptions. No situation is inherently positive or negative. How you view the world changes what you see in it. If you think negatively, you will see negativity in the world. Life satisfaction comes to those who pursue happiness and health, not those who deny realities that could lead to life satisfaction.

Those who deny reality do not see themselves as denying reality. To them, they believe in answers others do not accept. The answers are simple and based on their beliefs. Those who do not agree with them deny the beliefs they know to be true. Denying reality becomes a way of life. We learn things growing up that we initially question but give up asking about. We soon only accept information from people who we respect. The list of people who we respect becomes smaller until we only accept realities coinciding with our existing beliefs. An unquestioned belief is an unquestioned life. If your beliefs are unquestionable, you deny reality.

Dealing with reality without the shields of reality denial is difficult. We deny reality because we are uncomfortable with it. Denial is the first stage in dealing with grief and loss. Humans deny realities they dislike or are difficult to accept. We must accept the positive and negative aspects of reality. If you only accept what you perceive as positive, you are not accepting reality. Reality is full of death, inappropriate behavior, terminal illnesses, and ugly truths. Ignoring those ugly truths only makes them worse.

You must deal with all the horrible things that happen in life realistically. Your mental and physical health cannot hide from the reality you deny. Health problems you believe unrelated to your reality denial seem to develop from nothing. The health problems lead to injuries or more serious health problems. If you deny reality, you will not understand why this is happening. Hopefully, you can accept the reality of your serious health problems before they become fatal.

Some realities are invisible and easy to ignore. You can ignore the pain you live with daily because you do not see the pain. The pain can subside for a time and disappear from your consciousness. Eventually, the pain becomes a permanent part of your life. Emotional pain is even easier to ignore because we hide the cause of the pain. We separate the cause and effect in our mind. Emotionally abusive parents can be many times more damaging to a child than physically abusive ones. Both parents deny the reality of the damage they are doing to their children, but the emotional damage will last longer.

The biggest villains in fiction are the biggest reality deniers. None of them are happy or satisfied with their life, and most of them are unhealthy. They are under the mistaken impression that power and wealth are the only goals worth having. Happiness and health are only considerations when they interfere with their ability to gain more power or wealth.

The people we think of as villains never learned constructive ways of dealing with reality. They create their own realities and ignore the realities that impede their desires. They never truly get what they want, which is respect. Heroes get respect because they help other people and deserve respect. Villains get no respect because they do not deserve it.

Smart people are better at reality denial because they can think of more ways to deny reality. Sometimes their reality denial can appear as ignorance about an issue. The moment you call them ignorant, you are showing your ignorance of their point of view. Their opinion or belief originates from their denial of reality, but they are not ignorant. When dealing with people who deny reality, it is helpful to find a point of agreement so the conversation can continue. The conversation will develop over time and you can introduce your understanding of reality slowly. Declaring someone ignorant will only stop the conversation sooner.

One form of reality denial can show more reality denial. Denying the reality of your health will lead to you denying scientific realities. The scientific reality denial will lead to denying realities in your thinking, which will lead to not caring about other people. You can grow your reality acceptance just as you grew your reality denial. Our denial of reality comes from our beliefs. Our reality acceptance can only come from reality itself. Handling problems are easier when you are dealing with the actual problems and not what you believe are the problems. Viewing the world through your beliefs will blind you to the reality of the world.

You can only change the mind of others who deny major realities if you present a positive change to a subject in their focus area. If they focus on money, you must present a solution that benefits them economically. If they focus on religious beliefs, you must present a solution in line with their beliefs that benefits them. They ignore or deny reality presented outside what they accept as untrue. Reality denial is not a life sentence. We can change our ways and accept reality if others introduce it in ways we can accept. Most people's beliefs build over many years. Changing those beliefs will take time. If you care about them, the time is worth it.

There is no such thing as your reality or my reality. There is only reality. People say, "What if the green you see differs from the green I see?" That could be true if the other people were color blind, or we replaced their eyes with a cat's eyes. Human eyes are the same across all people. We can use green at stop lights because most people can see green, and they always put the green light at the bottom if someone is color blind. Your perception of reality does not change reality. There are no personal realities. Reality is the world as it is, not as you see it.

Reality denial in most societies becomes empowered by the leaders. We disseminate existing reality denial from above to those without power. The false reality spreads throughout the society and problems arise. All members of a society must accept the reality of the problems in the society before they can fix them. When only those without power are experiencing the problems, nothing changes. Most people in the society accept the false reality because they are unaware of the true reality.

Changes are necessary for a society to develop and handle problems inherent in advancements in technology and knowledge. Treating a society with the same rules and political structure as the past is not accepting the advancement of the society. We cannot compare the society in one location to a society in the same location from 100 years ago. The rules and political structure must represent the current inhabitants of the society. If they do not, the leaders of the society deny the current reality. Leaders encourage reality denial because they view reality acceptance as a threat to their power. The more a society accepts reality, the better it is for its citizens.

Change is not the only ingredient needed to encourage reality acceptance. Exchanging one reality denial for another will not improve your life and may make it worse. Only by accepting all of reality will you be able to deal with all problems. Any changes you make in your life before accepting and examining the reality of them will lead to unhelpful changes. Examining all the solutions to a problem requires a wide view of the problem. Changes made without this view will only lead to more problems.

Some realities are more complex than others. Accepting the realities of some problems may take time. The more time you spend examining a problem will result in better solutions. As you examine it, continue accepting new realities about it. The solution you reach based on reality will always improve your life. How much it improves depends on how much reality you examine and include in your solution. You must update solutions based on new realities that affect them. Time changes all problems to different problems.

Repetition is key to accepting and denying reality. The more you repeat either, the more you will accept or deny things in your life. Repeating reality accepting behaviors will allow you to continue to accept more reality. Repeating reality denying behaviors will allow you to continue to deny more realities. Developing a routine that encourages the acceptance of reality will improve your life. If you think negatively about something in your life, you are not accepting the reality of it. No realities are inherently positive or negative. Accepting realities you perceive as negative without preconceptions will allow you to see realities for what they are. Repeating a positive action will encourage you to accept positive actions from others.

If you deny more realities than you accept, you might be a reality denier. If you deny most realities, you are a reality denying expert. These experts can be dangerous to others. If they are leaders of a community, they can spread their message of reality denial to the entire community. With enough control over the community, they can create an entire reality denying society. When the entire community denies reality, it will spread to future generations, other communities, and to the world at large. Reality denial is bad for everyone.

Reality Blindness

Some people are reality blind. They either do not sense the reality or others have hidden the reality from them. A person who is blind is literally blind to the reality other people see. Other people can have weakened senses, limiting their ability to experience reality. Some people choose a limited ability to experience reality to shelter themselves off from it. When you rely on others to tell you about reality, you depend on those people. Depending on their grasp of reality, your view of it can become distorted. Your view of reality is in their hands.

Two people can be in the same room and perceive two distinct realities. We base much of what we perceive on our experiences. When you have no experience with certain types of people, you might have preconceived ideas about them. You will label anyone you meet as representative of an entire group of people. Most of these ideas will be incorrect because you base them on your beliefs. When others describe members of the group, they will seem like fictional characters. They are people we will never meet. Actually, you have met them, but you were blind to the reality of them as people.

Trauma can cause reality blindness. If you go through a life-changing or traumatic event, your mind may block these events from your conscious to avoid reliving the pain. This can be good for your health in the brief term. Dealing with these traumatic events will improve your view of reality in the long term. People cope with the traumas by developing rules for themselves, such as the rules for avoiding falling or a fire. These rules develop into unquestioned fears. If people continue to avoid examining traumatic events, they will remain blind to most realities.

Your perception of reality depends on how observant you are to the world. Some people focus only on a few aspects of reality to avoid dealing with others. Singularly focusing on one thing allows you to ignore or be blind to everything else. People with autism can focus so intently that they are blind to the emotions of other people. It may be obvious to one person, but is unseen, unheard, or unexperienced by another. The reality of the situation is the same, but the perception is different. A person with autism is not ignoring the emotions of others, they are blind to them. We should not punish others for being reality blind any more than a blind person who runs into another person. Recognizing reality blindness in yourself and others is a part of accepting reality.

Reality Accepting Exercise:

Notice the reality denial around you as you go through your day. Are people ignoring the world around them? How many inappropriate behaviors do you see? How many laws do people casually break? Do people make conscious decisions, or are they speeding through life automatically? Notice people who seem conscious of their happiness and health, if there are any.

Part 2
Health

Chapter 4

The Reality of Your Health

"There's nothing I can do about my health, and nobody lives forever. I'm going to do what I want until I die. People who talk about healthy living just want your money. Just because they say it will make you healthy doesn't mean I have to believe them."

Reality Denial

"When I eat healthy, exercise, and avoid stress, I feel my best. When I first started looking at my health, it seemed overwhelming. As I soon learned, it's just a matter of making healthy choices."

Reality Acceptance

The first and simplest concept of Reality Acceptance involves accepting the reality of your health. In today's world, it is no longer acceptable to be as healthy as average people. If you have no health problems, eat nutritious food, drink plenty of water, and exercise regularly, you are not average. An average person can have several health problems, eat high calorie meals at fast-food restaurants, drink excessive amounts of soda or coffee, and consider walking to his car as exercise. This trend is most distressing when you consider the number of health problems a person under age twenty can have. Accepting the reality of your health is easy, but changing your health for the better is not.

Some people care more about maintaining their car than they do about their health. The time they spend on their car never exceeds the time they spend on their body. If you drive your car to its limits without stopping, your car will breakdown. When your body breaks down, it is not as clear cut where the problem exists, and it may not be fixable. When you stress out your body or mind, you can permanently damage yourself. You can buy a replacement car if it stops operating, but the same is not true for your body and mind. Maintaining your health is much easier than fixing problems after they happen.

Advertisements have been lying to us all. Eating packaged food high in salt, sugar, and fat is unhealthy regardless of what commercials say. People believe words like organic, non-GMO, and natural are an assurance of healthy food. Natural foods do not require labeling as natural. Having a shopping list when you go to the grocery store is key to avoiding impulse buys. If you only have two days off a week from work, plan the five other meals you will eat at work. Instead of watching TV all day on your days off, look up recipes that are easy, healthy, and good tasting. Choose from healthy fruits and vegetables you know you enjoy. If you do not enjoy eating the healthy food, you will not eat it. Try other foods to see if you enjoy them. Eating healthy needs to become your main routine.

Mental and physical health closely relate to one another. You cannot have one without the other. When we ignore our health, we ignore reality. The side effects may include death. Your mental and physical health can cloud your perception of reality. People often have health problems because they are ignoring or denying the reality of their health. Your health problems will only get worse by ignoring them. If we do not understand the cause and effect of our health problems, we cannot fix them. Accepting your strengths and limitations is part of being a healthy person. Luckily, we have health professionals to help us become as healthy as we can. You must realistically examine and accept the reality of your mental and physical health to be your healthiest.

Some people think if they are physically fit, they do not have to worry about their mental health. Being physically fit will help your mental health, but you must have both to be a healthy person. Healthy emotions will help your mental health. Healthy behaviors will help your physical health. Your emotions can affect your physical health by interfering with physical activities. If you are too depressed to get out of bed, your physical health will suffer. Your activities can affect your mental health if you receive a physical injury that damages your brain. Being physically and mentally fit is mutually beneficial.

When I changed schools from elementary to junior high, all my close friends went to a different school. I found myself with no friends and little ability to make new friends. I focused on my schoolwork and got A's in all my classes. Every day I had days filled with bullies, kids ignoring me, and only being able to relate with adults. By the end of junior high, I was so miserable I thought about committing suicide. My focus was singularly on grades, while the rest of my life was empty. I was an ideal student, but a miserable person. My grades eventually declined, but my social life improved.

Social interactions can improve your health and help you live longer. Feeling lonely is one of the chief causes of depression. Interacting with others can keep you mentally fit, but not all social interactions are healthy. If your interactions center on unhealthy food and drinks, hostile conversations, and sitting for lengthy periods, the interaction is both physically and mentally unhealthy. We should only visit restaurants, bars, and nightclubs on special occasions. Friday night is not a special occasion. Interactions with others that are not mentally stimulating are an extra drain on your health when you add unhealthy activities. Unhealthy activities are unhealthy regardless of whether you enjoy the activities. The enjoyment is short-lived, but the unhealthy activities will damage your health in the long-term.

One aspect of our health many people forget is having a purpose in life. I have had several purposes throughout my life, but this book has been one of my primary interests and goals for the past few years. Aspirations, interests, and goals gives your life meaning. There is no inherent meaning to our lives, so it is up to us to create one. Some people have a purpose thrust upon them by others. It will not be meaningful to them if they are not interested in it. Without creating an interest or purpose for themselves, they will not aspire to do more than what other people told them to do. Feeling a lack of control in our lives is one of the major regrets we have when we look back on their lives.

Medical Experts

*"If you think I'm going to let some
doctors tell me what to do, you don't know
me very well. I know what my body needs.
Right now, it says I need a burger and fries
regardless of what those quack doctors
say."*

Reality Denial

*"I look to medical experts to tell me
what I may miss about my health. I would
rather visit them before I have a health
problem than after."*

Reality Acceptance

Medical experts can help us accept the realities we do not understand. Medical experts spend years developing the skills it takes to recognize medical issues. Trusting these experts is important to dealing with complex medical issues. The experts can only test you if technology will allow. You are the only one who can tell them how you feel. If you do not tell them about a pain or feeling inside you, they may not know it is there. Like a detective, they can only solve your medical issues based on clues they know about. Tell them everything you experience that is not normal.

Self-diagnosis is a skill. You can train yourself to diagnose your own simple medical issues. You cannot see a doctor and tell them to test you for everything that could be wrong with you. This is not a practical reality. You need to develop the skills to recognize the signs of your own distress. Some issues require medical experts to diagnose, but many issues are simple enough to diagnose on your own. Everyone should know their bodies and any abnormal problems they may be experiencing. When people are mentally and physically healthy, they only need to verify with a medical expert any abnormal symptoms which they do not understand.

Many people often ignore the advice of medical experts. We ignore unsolicited advice, no matter the source. People only seek advice from others when they have a problem. If they do not acknowledge they have a problem, the advice from experts will push them further away from examining the problem. Medical experts can only help others who want help. If people believe medical experts do not have their best interest in mind, they will ignore the advice from those experts. No medical experts will advise you to only listen to them and not consult other medical experts. Gather as much information as you can from as many sources as possible. Ignoring the same advice from multiple sources is ignoring reality.

Therapy

Reality Denial

Reality Acceptance

Therapists are medical experts who can help you recover from medical problems. The problems can be physical or mental. The therapist can help you deal with the reality of the issue or trauma you are recovering from. Therapy can only help those who will accept the help. A physical therapist helps you recover your physical movements to as normal as possible. A mental therapist helps you deal with emotional traumas or mental problems that may prevent you from having full mental health.

Physical therapy is necessary after an injury or other damage to your body. This can be from an accident or a muscle strain that develops slowly. The therapist may help you develop muscle building or stretching exercises to rehabilitate your body. The primary goal is to recover your movements so you can get back to a state before the damage occurred. It may not always be possible to return to your previous state. Limiting your movements is better than not moving at all. The physical therapy ensures you are in the best shape possible.

Psychologists and psychiatrists are the main mental therapists most people think about. Psychologists treat emotional and mental problems with behavioral interventions. Psychiatrists can prescribe medication and work on medication management. Other therapists include psychoanalysts, psychiatric nurses, psychotherapists, and several types of mental health counselors. Help is available to most people, but not all. If you have help available to you, use it when you need it.

A mental health therapist depends on gathering information about your emotions, behaviors, and other relevant facts to help them assess what type of therapy you need. We do not yet have the technology to understand someone's mental state beyond these outward signs. As with other medical experts, the more information they have, the better they can help. Therapists can suggest behavioral changes or other therapies to help you. They cannot help you if you do not tell them everything you are dealing with or you do not take their advice. The fundamental point of therapy is to allow you to understand your emotions and mental issues so you can improve your mental health.

We make amazing advances in physical and mental health therapies every year. These therapies help after a trauma has happened. Accepting reality can prevent most of these issues before they happen. By accepting the reality of your physical or mental health, you can solve minor problems before they become traumas. Denying the reality of minor issues will only allow those issues to grow worse. Therapy is an outside expert who can help you identify problems and solutions you may not know exist. If you could easily help yourself, you would have done so before. If you have a continuing health issue that is not improving, find the therapy that works for you.

SEE MORE EXAMPLES AT:

realityacceptance.com/category/health/therapy/

Reality Accepting Exercise:

Write a list of physical and mental health problems you have solved in your life. List the actions you took to fix those problems. Only focus on problems you actually fixed. Think of current problems with your health for which you are struggling. Are there any solutions from the past you could use on your current health problems? Were there resources you used in the past that could help you find help for your current problems?

Chapter 5

Physical Health

"I have problem knees, a torn shoulder, and I can't walk upstairs without pausing every few minutes. What can I do about it? The damage is done. Changing my habits now won't help."

Reality Denial

"I stretch every day, walk upstairs instead of taking an elevator, and exercise as much as I can. I feel better than most people my age and I've never had a major injury. Our bodies will treat us as well as we treat them."

Reality Acceptance

What Goes in Your Mouth

> *"I get plenty of nutrition in my diet.*
> *There are vegetables, protein, and bread*
> *in the hamburgers I eat. I drink soda all*
> *day, so I get more than enough water. I*
> *only have desert once a day, unless you*
> *count the energy bars I have for snacks*
> *throughout my day – which I don't."*

Reality Denial

> *"I started eating a vegan diet several*
> *years ago. I didn't know how good I could*
> *feel after eating. I thought heartburn and*
> *an upset stomach were just a part of*
> *eating. I have more energy, my weight is*
> *down, and my attitude has improved."*

Reality Acceptance

We have better working brains than ancient humans, but we use them to justify the illogical items we put in our mouths. Food is a social event, a status symbol, an art form, and a personal statement. We do not just eat to get rid of the pains within our stomachs; we eat to get rid of the pains within our hearts. I cannot say I have studied food and nutrition my entire life, but I have studied people. People search for meaning in everything, and food is no exception. They want their next meal to transform them into a superhero or transport them to the land of happy taste bud people. We oversimplify what we eat and drink. It is not a choice between something tasting good or being good for us. You can have both.

What you put in your mouth is a serious indicator of your health and longevity. Those people who say, "I don't want to live to be a hundred," are kidding themselves. Their hundred will take place at fifty. They will get the same aches and pains as the hundred-year-old whose body is twice as old. We cannot eat and drink unhealthy things most of our lives and be healthy. How something tastes is a minor part of why we eat. How food makes us feel is a much better measure of what we should eat. The person miserable after a high-calorie meal is the same person who raved about how good the food tasted while eating it. Food should not be a punishment or a reward, it should energize you.

I eat a mostly vegan diet. I eat meat, but it is rare. We often represent vegans as people out of touch with the evolution of humans. We were hunters and gatherers who ate meat, right? Humans are omnivores, but our Paleolithic ancestors ate little to no meat. If you genuinely want to eat like our ancient ancestors did, you will eat fruits, nuts, vegetables, and a minimal number of insects and small animals. Many people claim they need to eat meat as a source of protein. Protein gives you strength and is important for people to get it in their diet. Gorillas who are herbivores get plenty of protein from plants. The last time I checked, gorillas were much stronger than humans. Even the animals we eat get most of their protein from plants. Meat is not the only source of protein.

Restaurants, bars, grills, and nightclubs are not natural places to eat and drink. Humans spent millions of years without these places and only thousands of years with them. If most people eating and drinking in these places was healthy, I would call them mere advancements in how we eat. The reality is people eat and drink at these places because they are convenient, pleasurable, sociable, and fulfill individual cravings. People ignore the obesity, alcoholism, and multitude of health problems caused by eating at these places. If you only go to them on a special occasion, you will not experience health problems. If you go to them every day, you will have multiple health problems as you get older.

You do not know what you are putting in your mouth if you do not see it prepared. You rarely see your food prepared at a sit-down restaurant, from a pre-made meal, or from a fast-food restaurant. Preparing your own meal or seeing your meal prepared is the only way of knowing what is in your food. When we do not see our food prepared, the ingredients of the food become less important than how the food tastes. Eating only the best tasting foods can lead to a diet of junk food full of sugar, salt, and fat. These good tasting foods will lead to a shortened and painful death. Since you did not see the food made, your shortened and painful death may appear as standard aging. It is a sped-up aging that is unnecessary.

It is your choice to eat what you want. The only guidelines exist in your goals. If you want to be obese (said no one ever), eat whatever you are craving and ignore the ingredients. If you want to be healthy, eat healthy foods you enjoy eating. Avoiding looking at nutritional facts will not avoid the health consequences. Accept the reality of what goes into your mouth by knowing exactly what is in the food you eat. Do not hide the ingredients of the food you eat from yourself.

You put food in your mouth, but your stomach does the important job of digestion. You are feeding your stomach. Food spends a brief time in your mouth compared to your stomach and other organs. We should all please our stomachs more and our mouths less. We only notice our stomach when we have a problem with it. Pain is the quickest way to get you to think about what is in your stomach. If you have pain in your stomach regularly, change what you put in your mouth.

The part of food most people think about the least happens when we finish digesting it. It is a reality we are not eager to accept or examine, but it is important to our health. You cannot accept the reality of your digestion if you do not examine your urine and bowel movements. Before you freak out too much, I am only suggesting you notice irregularities and signs of problems. If you are not sure what is normal, consult health experts in person or online. Most of us do not talk about these things with others because they gross us out or make us uncomfortable. Being too embarrassed to talk about them could lead to many unhealthy consequences.

Before I finish talking about what we put in our mouths, I want to mention the importance of water. I had kidney stones at one point, so I know the problems from not getting enough of it. Water helps with hydration, digestion, circulation, and body temperature. You cannot be healthy if you do not drink enough water. Your body needs water all day. Remembering to drink throughout the day can be difficult if you are focusing on other things. Put water in your focus area or take water with you wherever you go. Forgetting to drink water is forgetting about your health.

Physical Exercise

*"I get plenty of exercise walking from
my car to my house. When I was younger, I
used to go to the gym all the time, but I
don't have time to go anymore. I also used
to do yard work, but I pay for someone to
do that now. I'm sure I'll exercise more
when I retire."*

Reality Denial

*"I try to exercise every day. No
matter where I'm at, I can always find
some physical activity to do. There's many
activities around the house that keep me
active and sweating. I don't need a gym to
move my body and workout my muscles."*

Reality Acceptance

Exercise is essential for maintaining your health. Some people naturally exercise by the lifestyle they live. Most of us rarely exercise our body throughout the day. It is wrong to think you are fine without exercising because you do not have any major health problems. Waiting for health problems is not an effective way to live. Incorporating exercise into your daily routine in important, regardless of your age.

My usual form of exercise is jogging and yoga. These exercises have come out of years of experimenting with various exercises to find what worked for me. The key to continuing to exercise was simplicity. I exercise at my house in the morning. I listen to podcasts and audio books as I exercise so my mind and body are getting a workout at the same time. Along with nutrition, exercise is important to living a long and healthy life.

You will be less likely to exercise the harder it is for you to exercise. People think they have to go to a gym to exercise. We can exercise at our house, near our house, or wherever we can move around and sweat. You must pick a time in your routine for exercising, start with simple exercises, and work your way up to more strenuous ones. If you do not enjoy your exercises, find exercises you will enjoy. Removing obstacles to exercising will ensure you continue to exercise.

We normally do not incorporate exercise into our routine when we are young because kids are naturally more energetic. Unfortunately, this is not true for all kids. If you grew up with parents who did not exercise, you will follow their example and not exercise in your adulthood. My dad naturally exercised by constantly working on physically taxing projects around the house. When he got older, he could no longer work on the projects and did not replace them with other forms of exercise. Near the end of his life, he developed many medical problems from this and other unhealthy habits.

Many people think playing sports is the same as exercising. People who play sports exercise so they can play sports and not hurt themselves. Sports are not a replacement for exercise. Sports without stretching and exercise can strain your body and cause injuries. We exercise to work out our muscles and joints in the most efficient manner. We should exercise our entire lives, but we can only play most sports for a limited time.

Avoiding pain is important to continuing to exercise. If you hurt or strain yourself exercising, you will use it as an excuse to stop. Start your day with stretching and well-rounded exercises. Your goal is to sweat. As you go throughout your day, choose to walk more, and take the stairs instead of an elevator. Try not to be sedentary for too long and drink as much water as you can. Exercise is the best way to ensure you remain physically fit. If you think you do not have time to exercise, today is the day to quit lying to yourself.

SEE MORE EXAMPLES AT:

realityacceptance.com/category/health/physical-exercise/

realityacceptance.com/category/health/physical-health/

Reality Accepting Exercise:

Plan a morning routine to start your day right. Find nutritious food to eat, choose exercises to get your body in motion, and ensure you get enough sleep the night before. This plan begins when you go to sleep the day before. Go to sleep with enough time to sleep as many hours as you need to feel rested. Know what you are going to eat the next day and know what exercises you can do in the time you have. The more you make it a habit, the more you can refine and improve your routine over time.

Chapter 6
Mental Health

"I work out at the gym because my job is so stressful. If I didn't have the job, I wouldn't be able to afford the gym. My wife is divorcing me because she says I'm always angry. Her loss. Of course, I might not be able to go to the gym anymore with what she's getting in the divorce."

Reality Denial

"I avoid stressful situations when I can. The stressful job I had was making me miserable. I've never been happier. I actively avoid stressful situations every day of my life."

Reality Acceptance

Happiness

"I don't have time to be happy. I have
bills to pay, kids to raise, and I'll never be
happy until I can afford the size boat that I
want. The only people who are happy are
too stupid to realize we weren't meant to
be happy."

Reality Denial

"I periodically check in with myself
and ask how satisfied I am with my life.
Happiness takes precedence over almost
everything else. I care about the happiness
of myself and the other people in my life."

Reality Acceptance

How happy you are will depend on your contentment and life-satisfaction. A content person is a person who recognizes happiness is worth having and cultivating. When we discourage children from experiencing happiness, they will grow up to be unhappy adults who spread their misery to others. Science, technology, and a general awareness of what creates happiness is allowing more people to be happy. We must accept the help to improve our happiness. It is important to avoid unnecessary activities that do not add to or detract from our happiness. Planning to be happy is important to being happy.

Pleasure is not happiness. Many things give you short-term pleasure such as sugar, drugs, alcohol, revenge, and getting away with a lie, but they are not happiness. Genuine happiness is a prolonged feeling permeating your life. It is a general life satisfaction. Long-term happiness takes years to attain and requires work to maintain. Happiness is as much a part of your health as exercise, eating right, and avoiding injuries. Thinking you are happy from short-term pleasures will not lead to genuine happiness.

Placing a smile on your face or pretending to laugh cannot force you into happiness. Happiness happens in your brain and not on your face. A true smile results from genuine happiness. I can always spot a fake smile. Happiness on the inside is more important than appearing happy. Being around others who are smiling and laughing can isolate you from them if you do not feel as they do. Smiling or laughing when you are not happy is lying to yourself and others.

Happiness is not a permanent state of being. It can come and go. No one will spend every waking moment in a state of bliss. You can only hope to fill a high percentage of your day with happiness. Believing you are happy differs from being happy. If you seek happiness throughout your day, you will find it. Happiness is more than satisfaction. Curiosity and excitement will also add to your happiness. Taking an active role in your happiness will allow it to grow.

Many businesses prey on those who seek pleasure and mistake it for happiness. Selling sugar water to massive amounts of people for huge profits is the perfect example of companies who sell pleasure while claiming their products create happiness. The sugar water will never give their customers anything beyond short-time pleasure and will negatively affect the health of their customers overall. I have no delusions that any company cares about their customers beyond profiting from them, but we should not accept the company's lies. They are peddling pleasure as a drug dealer does. The addiction to the product is the same goal for both businesses. The only difference is one business is illegal.

If you ignore the happiness of those around you, you will never truly be happy. Willful ignorance is ignorance. Happiness requires interacting with other people. Short-term pleasure is the most you can expect from ignoring those around you. Happiness comes from an understanding of what happiness truly means. Happiness is not ignoring the emotional states of others. Laughing at a funeral when no one else is laughing is an example of this ignorance. Comedians have to connect with crowds to make them laugh. If they ignore jokes that do not land with the audience, they will lose that audience.

Happiness requires laughing at your failures. Failing is a part of life. You will fail more than you succeed. When you fail, how you react can improve or worsen your happiness. Failure is humorous because you obviously did not intend to fail. Something went wrong. When I started accepting my failures and telling others about them, I could turn the failure into a humorous story. I was almost glad the failure happened so I could add to my happiness. Taking life too seriously will make you a humorless person.

Be the happiest person you know. Even though others may be happier than you, your goal should be to seek what truly makes you happy and endeavor to make others happy. Gathering happiness for yourself and those around you should be the goal for all of us. This may sound like a hippie-dippy thing to say (and it is), but it should be the goal of everyone who wants to live a content life. You are not competing with others to be the happiest. We can all be as happy as we are capable without detracting from others' happiness. We need to feel connected to other people. When we connect with others, we are happy. If you are not happy, you cannot help others become happy.

Happiness is the accumulation of fulfilled needs. These needs are mental. Some people think there is only one thing that can make them happy, but there are many things that make us happy. Losing one thing does not have to lead to losing your happiness. Many people are so accustomed to being miserable that a content person looks baffling to them. People will discourage you and try to make you as miserable as them. They are choosing to live a miserable life, but you do not have to make the same choice. Being where you want to be in life is the truest sense of happiness.

Feeling awe is a profound sense of happiness. It can be at a sunset, a natural wonder, or a beautiful moment you feel. If you are not happy in these moments, you will miss them. Noticing the feeling is just as important as noticing the beautiful moment. Not everyone feels a sense of awe at the same things. The feeling comes from novelty. If you see a beautiful sight every day, your sense of awe will diminish. Seeking new experiences will increase your chances of feeling awe and your overall happiness.

Emotions

*"I don't cry, I rarely laugh, and
anger is my main emotional outlet. Hating
others is the only way I know I have any
emotions at all."*

Reality Denial

*"Keeping in touch with my emotions
allows me to examine what areas in my life
need my attention. They let me know I am
human and connect me to other people."*

Reality Acceptance

There are no universal emotions, just like there are no universal languages. Every culture expresses their emotions differently. Some cultures have a cultural bias against expressing emotions. Emotional languages differ depending on the culture. Emotions in one culture may not exist in another culture, or another culture can interpret them differently. We learn about our own culture's emotions by observing others. The first emotions we observe come from our family. If your family does not have a healthy relationship with their emotions, you will struggle with yours. If an entire culture has unhealthy emotional relationships, you may never learn how to deal with your emotions properly. This emotional intelligence is important to learn if you want to be happy and healthy.

Parents can teach their kids to ignore their emotions through their actions or tell them directly to ignore or deny their emotions. If kids do not learn how to deal with their emotions, they may never learn to deal with them as an adult. Anxious children will grow up to be anxious adults unless they increase their emotional intelligence from an emotionally intelligent source. Finding a teacher of emotional intelligence may not be easy, but it is just as important as anything else we learn as we grow up.

When people misunderstand their emotions, their behavior will reflect it. Hate, revenge, depression, and anger become regular emotions, while happiness, elation, amusement, and awe become emotions they resent others for having. They use their negative emotions to focus their life on money, success, and power. This drive pushes others away from them. They may become successful but have no friends. With their social skills severely lacking, they do not value relationships with others.

Emotional intelligence is important to understanding our emotions and dealing with them. If we do not understand our own emotions, how can we understand someone else's? Part of developing social skills is dealing with our own and other people's emotions. If you grew up devaluing emotions, you may avoid emotions. Emotions are frustrating and uninteresting to you. You will misinterpret the emotions of others or ignore them completely. Emotional intelligence is a skill you must develop, or you will never be happy.

You will be better at sensing the emotions of people you know than strangers. We usually hide our emotions from strangers. Our emotional reactions come from our experiences with emotional events from our past. The more these emotional events are unexamined, the more extreme our emotions will become. Emotional people will have extremely positive and negative emotions. This is fine as long as you observe other people's emotions. Often, they do not see the emotions of others because they focus only on their own emotions. To deal with your own emotions, you must observe the emotions of others.

All emotions overlap with one another. People rarely experience only one emotion. Depression, anxiety, and fear can comprise several emotions and sub-emotions. Naming or labeling emotions is an oversimplification of the neurological processes involved in creating emotions. Pinpointing your emotions is not helping you deal with actual problems. Most emotions have a positive and negative possibility. We can re-categorize anxiety as excitement. We can re-categorize fear as anticipation. Writing your exact emotions is difficult and unnecessary. Understanding why you feel the emotions you do will increase your positive emotions.

Many of our emotional reactions come from our beliefs. If we believe the world is out to get us, we will feel negative toward it. The belief comes from our associations with negative emotions from the past. Removing our negative beliefs is necessary to deal with our negative emotions. The more we accept reality, the more we will seek positive emotions. These positive emotions will open us up to more positive realities.

Negative emotions come from realities you have not accepted. These realities can be losses, traumas, or other negative events that lead to anger, sadness, anxiety, or fear. The longer you have these negative emotions, the worse they will get. These negative emotions will manifest as negative behaviors. Treating the emotions or the behaviors will not help the problem. Your emotions do not come from single events. There may be a first event starting you on your negative path, but there are multiple causes of your negative emotions. Undealt with traumas will only add to your negative emotions. Dealing with your past traumas is essential for handling your negative emotions.

You should deal with each traumatic event separately. As you examine the negative events, you must remove your guilt about them. The trauma happened to you, so forgive yourself. The negative emotions come from your beliefs about these events. When you remove your guilt about these events, you will begin removing the negative emotions. It will not happen immediately, but the more you examine the reality of the events, you will feel the negative emotions disappearing.

Emotional pain develops into physical pain the longer we ignore it. You must accept the reality of your emotions or they will negatively affect your physical health. Suppressing your emotions can damage your heart, stomach, and brain. You may only notice the damage you have done to yourself when it is too late. Any physical pain that does not have a direct cause could be from emotional pain. Do not ignore your emotional pain or your health will suffer.

Suicide is an extreme example of ignoring or denying your emotional pain. How people commit suicide is not as important as why they do so. When our emotional pain is high, our emotional defenses are low. We will only see problems with no solutions and negative realities. A feeling of hopelessness fills our thoughts. We must create barriers for ourselves and others to prevent suicide. If you are in emotional pain, get help. Your emotional pain is much easier to deal with than your death.

Understanding your emotions is key to dealing with them. If you have no experience with examining your emotions, find a resource to better understand them. Negative emotions will only get worse the more you do not deal with them. Cultivating positive emotions is just as important as dealing with your negative ones. Ignoring or denying your emotions will ensure your life is miserable. Understanding your emotions is a big part of accepting reality.

SEE MORE EXAMPLES AT:

realityacceptance.com/category/health/emotions/

realityacceptance.com/category/health/mental-health/

Reality Accepting Exercise:

Think about things that take a toll on your mental health. Notice the people that stress you out, give you anxiety, or anger you. After those situations happen, think about them from the point of view of the other people involved in them. If they were happy and healthy, would they act as they did? Most of the time, they would not. Extend them the same empathy you would want if you were in their shoes. You can never know their motivations, but you can know they are dealing with many of the same mental health issues you and everyone else deal with. When you see people dealing badly with their mental health issues, learn from them.

Part 3
Knowledge

Chapter 7
The Reality of Your Knowledge

"I don't trust science or scientists. I don't believe they have our best interests in mind. They just make stuff up like everyone else, so why should I believe in them over what I can find out on the internet."

Reality Denial

"I look to science to give me the closest look at what we can really know. I understand the scientific method and know that if we do not follow it, we get scientific studies we can't replicate. Science has always got to be collaborative."

Reality Acceptance

Science is the best tool we have for examining reality and gaining knowledge. It comprises systematic methods of examining reality to understand it better. For that reason, many people avoid science. They may accept parts of science, but not all of science. Scientists represent people who seem hostile to their beliefs. Scientists present realities that go against what they hold to be true, whether those beliefs are religious, political, or cultural. Our beliefs are hostile to reality. They separate us from reality, while science brings us closer to it. Without understanding science, we cannot understand reality.

Collecting the perspectives of many scientists allows us to reach a consensus about reality. Science is an accumulation of knowledge, facts, and information we constantly question and never exempt from criticism. The scientific method and peer-reviewed studies ensure we have the most realistic examination of any subject. Science allows us to experience reality without filters. We can go beyond human perceptions, limitations, and biases to view a reality unseen except through the lens of science. Science has given us the most exciting view of reality and has advanced society well beyond our humble beginnings.

The three major branches of science are formal sciences, natural sciences, and social sciences. We can break each branch into many more specific branches, but, good news, I will not do that. We trace the beginnings of science back to Egyptian philosophers. Humans have been attempting to understand and study reality ever since we were conscious. We can only examine reality as snapshots of time, location, and motion. Reality changes over time, hampering our ability to study it. Studying reality in certain locations becomes problematic, if not impossible. Things in motion interfere with our ability to know if we are examining reality or an illusion. We must constantly update scientific information to better understand what we can know.

The basic building blocks of reality are atoms. From a scientific point of view, we only know atoms exist in theory. We cannot see atoms, but science has proven they exist through multiple experiments and studies. Reality comprises many things we can and cannot see, hear, touch, taste, or smell. In these cases, we need technology to help us sense what we cannot. All the significant advances in physical and mental health have come from scientific discoveries. Science has affected the lives of everyone living today. If you drive a vehicle, use a smart phone, survive a serious illness, or use the Internet, science has benefited you.

Scientists are reality detectives. They study past and present clues to solve the case of the reality they are examining. They piece together events from millions of years ago, recent findings, and collected data to form a complete picture of the crime scene of reality. We would still be in an age of ignorance without science. Most of what we know about the world comes from science. Even non-scientists can use the knowledge of science to better understand themselves and the world. We need not understand complex scientific concepts to understand science. A basic understanding of science is enough to accept the realities of our world.

The Scientific Method

*"The only thing I know about the
scientific method is that it's just another
set of rules that have no relevance in my
life. When they come up with a method for
making the best cheeseburger, I'll listen."*

Reality Denial

*"I'm not a scientist, but I use the
scientific method every day in my life. The
methodical logic of it can help me solve
any problem. If we can't prove something
with the scientific method, we cannot
currently prove it."*

Reality Acceptance

The scientific method is a method of gaining knowledge through a series of procedures and experiments to build our understanding of what we can know about reality. Bias and opinion can affect the results of a singular scientific study, but other scientists and scientific studies must independently verify each study. The scientific method is not about one scientist or group of scientists. It is about developing a repeatable method of testing a hypothesis. Consistency is important in scientific experiments and in the scientific method.

Basic Steps of the Scientific Method:

- Ask a question.

- Conduct background research.

- Construct a hypothesis.

- Test the hypothesis with experiments.

- Analyze the data.

- Form a conclusion and publish the results.

Scientists repeat these steps several times before a scientific study reaches a conclusion. They test and retest theories to find conclusive data. They publish the resulting data in peer reviewed scientific journals. Other scientists conduct more studies on the same subject and hopefully reach a scientific consensus. If they do not reach a consensus, they conduct more scientific studies. Even when they reach a scientific consensus, scientists and scientific groups will continue to expand upon our understanding of the subject. When they prove the theory with several independent studies, the theory can become knowledge other scientists can build on. The proceeding was a gross oversimplification of the scientific method. If it interests you to learning more, go with that interest.

The news often comments on individual scientific studies, creating sensational news headlines. This is a misunderstanding of what individual studies represent. Unless you take the time to examine the results of a scientific study completely, you will not understand what the study is saying. People uninvolved with the study often write sensational headlines. Most times, the actual study only changes our understanding of a subject, but the news headline declares a revolutionary advancement or tragic finding. Science is under the same economic restraints as the news. Scientific studies can be expensive, and scientists must prove the studies are worth the cost. It is not the best system, but it allows scientists to conduct further studies to advance our knowledge.

Time is important in the scientific method. You cannot remove steps or speed up results in science. When people complain pharmaceuticals take too long to come to market, they are misunderstanding the scientific method. Thoroughly testing pharmaceuticals takes time. They must test the promises and side effects to ensure the safety of every drug. The scientific method, slow as it is, is what ensures our safety. Not taking the time to test drugs properly can lead to harmful consequences.

Scientists must deal with enormous time spans when practicing the scientific method. The Earth formed about 4.54 billion years ago. Humans appeared about 200,000 years ago. The scientific method has only been around about 800 years. We have only had 800 years of scientific study to analyze the information we have gathered. We use carbon dating and other scientific methods to analyze the information and continue making new discoveries. The scientific method ensures we can reliably compare the information we have gathered with our current understandings of science.

The scientific method is the most fundamental concept in science. We can understand reality more by building on our knowledge of it. Doubting scientific knowledge differs from doubting someone's opinions or beliefs. We must understand a scientific concept to disagree with it. The scientific method is one of the greatest inventions humanity has produced. It allows scientists from all over the world to compare reliable results and share their knowledge with one another.

Evolution

Reality Denial

Reality Acceptance

Did humans evolve so we could type on a computer, drive cars, or land on the moon? Evolution is a process that developed over millions of years. Humans ascribe our own purposes to ourselves and other species because we see our lives as purpose driven. We are not born with these purposes any more than we are born with knowledge. People reject evolution because it is complex and still misunderstood even by scientists. It is millions of years of history we only began studying about 800 years ago.

Evolution is a natural process of ensuring future generations are better able to survive and adapt. If you can adapt to a changing world, your species will live on. Gigantic animals such as dinosaurs could not adapt to a world without enough resources for them. Animals at the top of the food chain depend on abundant sources of food. Evolution ensures one species does not overly dominate over other species. The extinction of a species comes when they cannot adapt to changes.

The most adaptive species are scavengers. They have become more adaptive to competing with other scavengers. This adaptability of their brains has increased in efficiency generation after generation. The ultimate scavengers are humans. Our physical imperfections were more than made up for with the efficiency of our brains. We were not the biggest, fastest, strongest, or most armored animals, but we used our brains to overcome those deficiencies. Humans adapted to multiple environments to thrive around the world.

Studying evolution in science meant humans could see their place among all living species. This information has been the greatest asset of humanity. We could study ourselves and other species to better understand the world. Some people used their brains to expand our understanding of the world, while others used their brains to control other people, suppress information, and ensure humanity would be its own worst enemy.

People who ignored or denied the evolutionary lessons of science saw themselves as superior to other species. They exploited scientific knowledge that benefited them and ignored what did not. Science and evolution were things they believed in or they did not. It was not a tool they used to understand the world; it was a tool they used to prove their superiority. They used technological advances developed by scientists to dominate other species. This domination caused the extinction of many species and could cause the extinction of humans.

Reality Accepting Exercise:

Think of a scientific topic you are interested in. It can be space, evolution, environmental studies, psychology, or any subject you can scientifically study. What are the scientific methods they could have used to study it? Think of all the factors they used to study it. How many unusual places, environments, people, instruments, and points of view did they collect to reach a scientific consensus?

Chapter 8
Knowledge, Information, and Facts

"How can we truly ever know anything? Your facts are not my facts. By the time you learn information, it's outdated. If the internet has taught me anything, it's facts change like the channels on my TV."

Reality Denial

"Basic facts change little over time. We add information other information and expand our knowledge of everything. Our experiences and beliefs influence our interpretation of facts, but the facts are the same. We can only hope to discover them."

Reality Acceptance

Language and writing were important steps in the evolution of humans. When information could travel to other locations and other times, the world could connect as a whole. The printing press, computers, and internet advanced the dissemination of information even further. We can and should share information so others can build upon it. Knowledge is neither positive nor negative for the world. It is what we do with our knowledge that determines our future.

Governments and other world powers have tried to suppress information, but they always fail. With time, the ease with which we can know information is growing. The more freedom disseminates the world, the more knowledge people can freely know. The more people know about the world, the more humanity benefits. Knowledge about the world brings us closer to understanding reality and improving life for everyone.

Knowing a fact differs from understanding it. Memorizing facts is not knowledge about those facts. The facts are useless until we know why those facts are important. Receiving the same facts from multiple sources in unique ways will reinforce them. We reinforce information and misinformation with repetition. We view reality through what we know or think we know. Accepting or denying reality will increase as we get older. The more our experiences coincide with our knowledge, the more we will believe our knowledge is factual. This can be a problem if our sources of information are not diverse.

Facts can impede our ability to accept reality. When people focus on facts alone, they ignore the complete reality of situations. A general understanding of a situation is much more important than specific facts about it. We can misunderstand, misuse, or deny facts to misinterpret the situation. Focusing only on the validity of facts will lead to ignoring simple realities and leave us only accepting facts with which we already agree. We should collect facts to understand a situation, not to describe it.

Some people mistake facts for answers and cling to them personally. If we are only looking for answers, we will only find simple ones. Facts only answer specific questions, rarely answer meaningful questions, and are sometimes irrelevant. If you focus only on the facts, you miss many underlying realities. Arguing over irrelevant facts will ignore relevant ones. We must search for relevant factors and clues to answer meaningful questions. Receive all the information you can and ignore irrelevant facts.

People who think they have all the answers have accepted simple answers and stopped asking questions. Confronting their answers is confronting them as people. Holding on to unchanging answers will lead to an outdated view of the world. When the scientific community downgraded Pluto to a dwarf planet, people took it personally. They would have to change what they knew about the Solar System. The scientific community was only correcting an incorrect answer scientists had long accepted as factual. The answers we think we know should always be questionable.

Subject experts accept the facts of a subject and accept those facts will change. The subject interests them, not the facts about the subject. Facts that change represent the most exciting facts for experts. They increase their understanding of the subject and their interest in it. We turn to experts to interpret facts for this reason. Experts can separate relevant from irrelevant information. Facts only create a snapshot of a subject. Experts study subjects over time because facts change with time. We need experts for reliable interpretations of facts.

Information is only as reliable as its source. Researching the source of the information is just as important as researching the information. If the information comes from a questionable source, it is less reliable and useful. Knowledge from an expert or expert publication is the most useful information. When you find a reliable source of information, use it when considering other sources. You can use various sources to verify the legitimacy of individual sources. The more a source agrees with others, the more you can trust it. If you accept all information, you will fill your head with misinformation. Finding reliable sources is key to finding reliable information.

You should always be skeptical of information only coming from one source. The same information from several independent resources is more reliable. Rumors and gossip usually originate from one source. We should be skeptical of all information, especially if it contradicts other sources. News outlets often have single sources for information, making them unreliable as a source. When you let one resource dictate your knowledge, your knowledge is unreliable.

The human brain can only keep so much information. If you try to keep too much, you will overload it. This could be as simple as not remembering the information or not being able to focus on other parts of your life. Your social interactions, daily tasks, common sense, and problem-solving skills will suffer. A computer can handle storing vast amounts of information because the computer does not have to worry about human bodily functions. Overloading yourself with information will drain your basic human functions. People who can remember vast amounts of information can often do little else. Valuing information over everything else will lead to a negative and indifferent view of life.

Knowledge, information, and facts are all important to understanding reality. If we only have our individual experiences for viewing reality, we will limit our view of it. The more knowledge we have as a global community, the better we can understand reality. Most of the verifiable facts and information we have about the world comes from science. The scientific community uses the scientific method to insure they are a reliable source of information. The more we learn about reality, the more we realize how much more there is to learn.

SEE MORE EXAMPLES AT:
realityacceptance.com/category/knowledge/information-facts/

Reality Accepting Exercise:

Think about a subject you have a great deal of knowledge about. Write all the facts and information you can think of. Look at each of the facts or pieces of information. Take each of the facts and verify the authenticity of those facts with multiple evidence-based sources. Was what you wrote complete and accurate with each of the sources? Were there contradictory facts among the various sources? Did you learn additional facts you did not know? As you dig deeper into the subject, you will find more information that uncovers even deeper dives into it. The only limit to how much information you can take in is your interest in the subject.

Chapter 9
Learning from Our Failures

*"I have had very few failures in my
life. Failure is an option that I don't
accept. I do whatever it takes to get the job
done. If that means covering up my
failures, so be it."*

Reality Denial

*"I have failed often in my life, but I
learned from every single failure. It's only
a failure if you continue to do things that
have proven ineffective in the past. I try
not to make the same mistake twice."*

Reality Acceptance

Much of learning in science is learning from our failures. We learn more from failures than we do from successes. Failures teach us how we learn. The information we learn from scientists and other educators results from many failures and a few successes. Learning information without learning how we attained the information makes it less interesting. We cannot learn from information without understanding the context of how we originally learned it. Understanding how to deal with incorrect information teaches us how to find correct information. It also teaches us how we learn. Knowing how we learn will help the quality of our learning.

People must learn language, speech, driving, and any skill from others. We first learn from our parents, siblings, and other family members. Eventually, we learn from our teachers, friends, neighbors, and a host of other people. Most of the information is simple at first, but gets more complex. Your parents may hold back certain topics from you such as death, because it is not a simple concept to explain to a child. How you learn becomes more complex as you learn more information. You will prefer certain learning styles, but the more learning styles you encounter, the better you will learn.

Some people are afraid of knowledge and discourage others from learning. Being afraid of knowledge is being afraid of reality. There is no dangerous knowledge. Even a grim truth is important to learn about preventing future grim truths. Learning from the mistakes of the past is important for everyone. You should value your failures. If you deny your failures to yourself or others, you have not learned from them. Presenting only your best face to the world will devalue your life. Learning the ugly truth about it allows you to improve your future.

SEE MORE EXAMPLES AT:
realityacceptance.com/category/knowledge/learning/
realityacceptance.com/category/knowledge/learning-from-failures/

Rewards and Punishments

Reality Denial

Reality Acceptance

Rewards are just as bad as punishments for learning a lesson.
Both originated from the simplistic thinking of right and
wrong we learned as kids. People learn how to get rewarded
and avoid punishments without learning from their actions.
We reward students with good grades and punish them with
poor grades, but do not care if they are learning. We lock
schools into a grading system, which advances students good
at taking tests. Sometimes, they must lower the standards of
the tests so more students can pass. Learning from incorrect
answers is more important than focusing only on correct
answers.

We dispense most rewards and punishments inappropriately and illogically. We reward one person for being born into wealth and punish another for being born into poverty. Allowing one person to have billions, while most people struggle to get by, is illogical and unethical. The competitive thinking of most societies allows these discrepancies to happen. If the world only punishes you, you will do whatever it takes to reap rewards wherever and however you can. Laws, rules, and the judgments of others do not matter as much as achieving the rewards you have only seen or heard about. Anything is better than the constant punishment of your life. The reality of the rewards you seek will never live up to your expectations.

Imprisonment, torture, and other forms of punishment do not work. Accepting reality, rehabilitation, and other forms of learning will work. To change people's behavior, you must change their thinking and beliefs. If they believe you will not punish their inappropriate behavior, it will continue. They will ignore all punishments because all of them are arbitrary. Learning from our inappropriate behavior will only happen if we accept the reality of our behavior. We can only teach those who will learn. Punishment will ensure their behavior gets worse.

Rewards recognizing the wrong things are just as ineffectual as punishments. Rewarding one person who is slightly better than other people in a competition is punishing most of the people. Recognition for improvement, overcoming an obstacle, or demanding work will encourage us to continue learning and growing as people. Most of the reward we receive from accomplishing a task happens while we are accomplishing it. Any outside rewards we receive afterward are minor compared to the lessons we learned.

SEE MORE EXAMPLES AT:
realityacceptance.com/category/knowledge/rewards-and-punishments/

Reality Accepting Exercise:

Think about a time they punished you as a child. For some of us, this will not be difficult except for choosing only one. After your punishment, were you ever punished again for the same thing? Were your punishments always the same, or did they vary based on the infraction? Looking back on them, do you think they were affective in changing your behavior? Were your siblings, friends, or classmates punished more or less than you? Did the amount they punished any of you make you a better person? We tell ourselves that punishing kids will make them better people, but there are plenty of unhappy and unhealthy adults who only learned how to avoid repercussions as kids. We teach negative behavior through negative reinforcements.

Chapter 10
Logic and Planning

Logical Thinking

"I try to do things logically, but I always have problems with other people. I don't know why they can't see the logic in what I'm doing. It makes sense to me. They must be stupid."

Reality Denial

"If I'm doing something that makes little sense to other people, I must not be doing it in the most logical way. I always take input from others so I can learn better ways of doing things. What seems logical to you is not always the most logical answer."

Reality Acceptance

Understanding how logic works is part of being logical. You cannot apply logic narrowly. If something is logical to you but no one else, it is not logical. Logic does not have ethics, psychic abilities, or unquestionable facts. It is a thought process based on analyzing all available data and choosing the best option for all involved. Understanding logic is key to understanding life and being happy. If you see the world as a big, illogical mess, your life will become a mess. When you look at the world logically, you will see order in what you thought was chaos.

Things that appear logical to one person are not necessarily logical for everyone. Logic is interactive. Actions are logical when they interact logically with other people. Using logic is like developing code for a computer program. The more information (data) you have, the more logical your decisions are. Your solutions will be more logical the more factors you include in your analysis of a problem. Making a logical decision includes your experiences with the problem. If you do not have enough information or experience with a problem to make a logical decision, wait until you do.

You can only make logical decisions by accepting the reality of a problem. We decide how to solve a problem by thinking about the past, present, and future of it. We must research the problem's past, observe the current situation, and plan solutions for it. Decisions based on irrelevant or arbitrary information will be illogical. We must balance logic, emotions, and practical concerns. Logical arguments without limits will lead to unbalanced and illogical decisions. Problem solving always involves change. If you or others are unwilling to change, the problem will not get solved.

You can question other's decisions only if you have knowledge of how they made their decision. Otherwise, you are speaking from an uninformed opinion. Assuming others made arbitrary decisions is not respecting them. Decisions you do not understand are not illogical decisions. When we criticize others for their decisions with little knowledge, we usually do so without them being present. If they were present, we would not be so quick to judge them. We get subconsciously embarrassed by our misunderstanding of their decisions.

I am fascinated by illogical behavior. People focus so much on their inner goals and ignore the larger picture of the world around them. They do not accept the complete reality of the situation and behave illogically. If we narrowly focus on a few factors relevant to a singular goal, we will ignore other factors and people. Illogical decisions are usually short sited. We might take one step forward and three steps back because we are ignoring the larger picture. Quick decisions are always illogical decisions. We must quickly determine the reality of the situation based on little information.

Logical behavior is only logical if we base it on all available information. Ignoring information around us will lead to illogical behavior. Risk takers will ignore the danger of a situation. Denying information around us will lead to inappropriate behavior. Self-centered people will deny their effect on others. Doing only what is logical for you does not consider other people. If your behavior is illogical around other people, it is inappropriate behavior. Logical behavior is appropriate behavior. We can never apply logic narrowly.

We will break illogical laws and rules. Following illogical rules is illogical behavior. Inadequate rules do not deal with all the realities of the behavior they are trying to change. Laws and rules should never be permanent. We should base them on current information and add to them with additional information. The more difficult it is for laws to change, the more outdated and illogical they will become. A law only benefiting a certain segment of society is illogical and unethical. Breaking illogical rules and laws is inevitable.

Teach people logic, and they can learn anything. I can fix my shower because I can logically figure out what to do to fix it. Logic is the key to learning. If you see the logic of a lesson, it will be easier to learn. When you take a test, do not give the answer you think is correct. Give the answer you think the test maker wants to see. The order you learn something matters less than understanding the logic of what you learned. We can look up a lost or forgotten step, but we must understand the logic of the steps.

Planning for the Future

"I like to be spontaneous and often start projects before I know what I'm doing. Redoing things or not finishing most of them is just how I like it. I just do what I want and hope it works out."

Reality Denial

"I never do something without having a plan in mind. Being halfway through doing something and finding out I should have done it differently distresses me. It's not fun finding out you wasted hours of your day."

Reality Acceptance

Scientists must constantly plan for the future. They must plan experiments, make predictions, and use their time wisely. They must carry many scientific studies out with limited time, space, and resources. If they do not plan well, they will be a waste of the time, space, and resources. We can learn from science by planning for our own futures. As with science, we cannot plan for the future if we do not understand the present.

Thinking about something before it happens can prevent many future mistakes. Some people ignore the reality of situations by only thinking about the present. Giving no thought to your future is ignoring it. Planning is merely thinking about future actions and preventing future problems. Instead of making a series of last-minute decisions, you plan your actions to avoid preventable problems. If you are rushing through life, you are barely thinking about the present. You will make quick and unplanned decisions that will lead to more problems.

Planning does not ignore your present life. Your experiences in the present and past inform your decisions about the future. How well you plan your future depends on your knowledge of current realities. If you are unsure of your plans for the future, you need to research the possibilities. You can only deal with difficult possibilities if you understand what those possibilities are. Planning for unlikely possibilities will detract from the likely ones. Having multiple plans will increase your chances of future success.

Accept the reality of your future by planning for it. There are many ways to get the same result. Do not pin your plans to one possibility. Expecting a specific result will always lead to disappointment. When you are executing your plan, let reality guide you to the next step. Accept barriers as problems you need to handle before you continue toward your goal. Planning your future success or avoiding future problems is an excellent use of your time in the present.

SEE MORE EXAMPLES AT:
realityacceptance.com/category/knowledge/planning/

Reality Accepting Exercise:

Think about a future plan you have only talked about with others, but have not fully developed. Write any barriers to that plan you can think of. For each barrier, write several solutions for each one that could deal with or eliminate it. Planning a future with only one trajectory for getting there is not really planning. A plan must involve solutions for as many future problems and barriers as you can imagine.

Chapter 11
Complex Realities

"I like simple things. If something looks complex, I'm not interested in it. My life is too busy to worry about dealing with complex things. I'm just a simple person I guess."

Reality Denial

"I know that life comprises complex realities, but most of them don't change my day-to-day living. They are points of interest for me. If life were simple, it would be boring. I'm never bored in this gloriously complex world."

Reality Acceptance

Understanding complex realities is important in science. The more you examine something, the more complex it appears. We do not require non-scientists to examine or understand complex realities. Most scientists find complexities exhilarating, but most non-scientists find them confusing and boring. Complex realities exist in ecosystems, mathematics, technology, and anywhere we must consider an enormous number of factors to understand something. We need not understand them individually, but they are crucial to examine for humanity.

Most people avoid complex realities because they cannot understand them easily. We have enough going on in our lives without examining vast amounts of information and only understanding a portion of it. People do not reap vast rewards for most examinations of complex realities. In fact, complex discoveries often go unnoticed by most people. When we have a challenging time accepting basic realities, we will not accept complex realities. Some people reject these realities because they like simple answers. Complex realities do not have simple answers.

The reason people examine complex realities is the same reason people enjoy solving more complex puzzles as they get older. Challenging our minds is an important part of our mental health. If you only challenge yourself to a certain level, you will never grow beyond it. At this point in human history, complex realities are the only realities we have yet to figure out. Scientists all over the world have examined realities from different perspectives and compared their findings with one another. The only reason the world does not agree on these basic scientific facts is scientists do not populate the world.

People who accept simple answers to complex questions are people who do not ask complex questions. Complex realities only come with complex answers. To find them, you must ask complex questions. If you avoid complex questions, you are avoiding the most interesting parts of reality. Complex stories are more satisfying to watch because they encompass multiple stories that must connect at the end. When people describe others as simple-minded, they are not paying them a compliment. Understanding complex realities will not make everyone happier, but understanding basic realities will.

Numbers and Mathematics

*"I never did well in math. I just find it
boring and not relevant to my life. The
only numbers I care about are picking the
right lottery numbers so I can quit my
job."*

Reality Denial

*"I use mathematics all the time. When
I hear people say they don't need to
understand mathematics, I'm surprised. I
don't know how these people pay for
anything, build something, or balance
their checkbook. I'm glad I'm not their
accountant."*

Reality Acceptance

Numbers permeate our lives. Most people have a basic
understanding of mathematics that does not include statistics.
They speed on the freeway in the fast lane one car length away
from the car in front of them, but freak out if they have to ride
in a plane. They will use homeopathic "medicine" that will at
most do nothing for their health. Understanding probability
and complex numbers is not in most people's knowledge base,
but it should be. It only takes a bit of work to understand the
basics of mathematics.

Many people have problems dealing with astronomically
large numbers. They can handle hearing about or even
picturing a million of something. When you get to a billion
and beyond, our minds have a harder time comprehending
such large numbers. Infinitely small numbers are equally

complex and difficult to comprehend. Finding relative points in comparing complex numbers is helpful. Comparing astronomical distances to distances you understand allows you to picture their sizes relative to one another. We compare the planets in the solar system by their distance from the sun and size relative to the Earth.

Comparing an atom to the size of the universe is an example of comparing large numbers to small numbers. An atom is so small that classic physics could not describe them. The universe is so expansive that humans will never observe most of it. These two extremes point out the differences in scale scientists must consider. Fortunately, a non-scientist does not have to worry about these extremes. Most people can handle everyday mathematics, but they claim otherwise.

The metric system is an international system of measurement. Scientists use the system around the world to measure weight, mass, distance, height, speed, and volume. Britain and the United States have not widely adopted the metric system. This has more to do with the political powers in these areas than logical scientific reasoning. The universal measuring system allows scientists around the world to conduct experiments with numbers they can compare reliably with other scientists. Mathematics is a universal language that connects the world like no other.

We use numbers to make predictions about the future. Predicting the likelihood of future events is based on percentage changes of events. We use numbers to count specific types of cells in our bodies, observable black holes in space, and anything we want to compare to something else. These counts are simplistic uses of mathematics. Comparing the number of objects, interactions, or living beings allows scientists a wider view of reality. As the world changes, so must the numbers. We use percentages and other mathematical principals to better our predictions of the future and our future itself.

Understanding the probability of something is not as difficult as most people think. Odds of a million to one is 0.01%. Essentially, it is 0%. The chances of winning the lottery are about 13 million to one. Again, that is essentially 0%. You win lower amounts if you get some numbers, but you still only have about 17 to 1 odds of winning anything. I no longer want to win the lottery because I would rather earn the money. Wishing for something and beating the odds is not earning the money. If you are born into a family with money, you have again not earned the money. Understanding probability allows you more predictable results.

Some people use misunderstandings in mathematics to convince others of false realities. People make many predictions about the future, but only focus on the times they were correct in their predictions. These people are no more psychic than people who play the lottery for years and finally win. Most scams for money are playing on the ignorance of scammed individuals. If you do not understand the mathematics involved in an investment, do not invest in it. The best thing we can do is educate victims so they can avoid being victims again.

We cannot make personal predictions using general social predictions. A societal trend will not inform you about specific individuals in the society. If you know you are more likely to get into an accident near your house, you should not feel safer driving on the freeway. The only reason accidents occur near your house is because that is where you are most of the time. You may go to separate places in a day, but you are likely to leave and come back to your house several times. Societal predictions are only helpful to predict societal trends.

Mathematics has advanced our understanding of the world more than any other form of communication. If you understand mathematics, you can understand most of reality. You can confuse people by mistranslating most languages, but you can only misunderstand mathematics or get it wrong. Many people avoid understanding mathematics and other sciences because of the rigidity built into them. Mathematical concepts build upon one another. If you misunderstand basic concepts, you will never understand more complex ones. Mathematics is one of the greatest scientific tools used to understand reality. We can all use mathematics to understand reality better.

Reality Accepting Exercise:

Think about a complex subject that you do not completely understand. Are you interested in that subject? Is it relevant to your everyday life? Do you understand parts of it, but do not understand it as a whole? Do you understand the basics of it, but do not understand specific parts of it? Write a list of anything you do not understand about it. Take each item on the list and look for answers to each one. The more individual items you understand, the more the whole subject will come into focus.

Part 4
Thinking

Chapter 12

The Reality of Your Thinking

"I hate to lose. Losing is for losers. Winning is everything! I do everything I can to make sure I'm a winner. Winners have everything and losers have nothing."

Reality Denial

"We cannot have all of something or nothing at all of it. You can get 100% on a test, but life doesn't work that way. We speak in terms of good or bad, but at no point is something all good or all bad. We live our lives in the middle of these two extremes."

Reality Acceptance

There is a close relationship between the way you think and your mental health. I debated what to include here and in the mental health section of this book. Examining our thinking is complex and has developed through many scientific fields. Philosophers, neurologists, psychologists, and many other experts have struggled to find why we think as we do. Much of the reality of our thinking is a mystery to ourselves, other people, and humanity. Accepting the reality of your own thinking will help you understand why others think as they do. Avoiding negative emotions is about avoiding negative thinking.

Humans are adept at thinking. Using our brains is how we decide, take actions, and stay alive. Many animals are bigger, stronger, and have larger teeth, but humans can think themselves out of an attack or into a meal to eat with their small teeth. Human beings have come so far that we now think about thinking. We wonder about things and seek knowledge, but we also hate ourselves and deny the realities we do not want to accept. The brain can do as much good as it can harm us. Our perceptions, beliefs, and clouded judgment can allow our brains to accept a mistaken reality. Our brains are powerful tools, but they have limits.

Thinking is not linear, even though dreams lead us to believe they are. Dreams happen concurrently, whereas most thoughts do not. You get vague flashes of images, words, and connections. It may be possible to experience someone else's thoughts someday, but it will be flashes of seemingly unrelated images, memories, and partial sentences. A poorly organized collage is the closest thing to picturing how our thoughts might look. Your brain is gaining memories, feelings, and emotions when you are thinking of solving problems, making decisions, avoiding pain, and staying alive. Understanding these processes is far from simple, but necessary if we want to understand how our minds work.

Thinking leads to interest. Interest leads to knowledge. Knowledge leads to solutions. Outside forces influence your thoughts, interests, knowledge, and problem-solving skills. When those influences are negative, extreme, or factually deficient, they will negatively influence your thinking.

Independent thinking is a skill that can save you from these outside influences. Complete independent thinking, however, can lead to a self-centered form of thinking that will isolate you from others. Finding positive influences on your thinking will help you form positive ways of thinking.

Some people can develop a fear of what others think, or even their own thoughts. The fear is highest when we are talking to strangers. They are new and, therefore, unknown to us. The ambiguity causes us anxiety and a host of other emotions. We get excited about positive experiences we suspect will make us happy, but we find an unknown experience anxiety provoking. This fear of the unknown can lead to people only experiencing things with which they are familiar and avoiding novel experiences or other people. The people currently in your life are the only people you interact with or exchange thoughts. Eventually, you think the same thoughts they do and avoid thoughts that contradict what you already believe.

Nuanced thinking is a reality accepting way of thinking. Developing a nuanced way of thinking takes years to develop. Some people never gain this skill and remain in an extreme pattern of thinking their entire lives. The result of thinking this way is dying bitter and alone. When your thinking is more nuanced, you accept the reality that few things in life have simple answers. As a public service announcement, I feel it necessary to tell you this way of thinking will disturb people in your life who are extreme thinkers. Nuanced thinking is a threat to their all-or-nothing thinking. If you have friends who think only in extremes, you may want to re-think those friendships.

Your thinking has as much, if not more, to do with your health as your physical and mental health. If you base your actions on your beliefs and not actual knowledge, you will misinterpret the world. These beliefs will heavily influence your perception of the world. Avoiding this negative thinking is a matter of learning about the reality of the world rather than believing it is unavoidably stressful and negative. How you think about the world affects the quality of your life and the people in your life.

SEE MORE EXAMPLES AT:

realityacceptance.com/category/thinking/

Beliefs

*"My beliefs are sacred to me. If you
disagree with my beliefs, you disagree with
me. I have a tough time dealing with
people who don't believe as I do, so I stay
away from them."*

Reality Denial

*"I consider beliefs to be temporary
guesses about the world. Most of the
beliefs I've had in my life were wrong. I'd
rather know something rather than believe
it."*

Reality Acceptance

Beliefs are not inherently positive or negative. The beliefs will
not hurt or improve your life. It is only when your beliefs
cloud your view of reality, they can harm you. If you believe
someone is trying to hurt you when they are trying to help
you, your beliefs are harming your quality of life. When you
base your beliefs on solid evidence and sound reasoning, you
are still only making an educated guess. What you believe
about reality will hinder your view of it. If you observe
something with preconceived notions, you only perceive that
with which you agree. You are observing the scene as a biased
witness. Belief is simple, but reality is complex. Your beliefs
are clouding your view of reality. Reality does not change
based on your beliefs, but your beliefs should change based on
reality.

Beliefs should never be permanent. Having beliefs you
carry with you for years will only shelter you from reality. We

should base our beliefs on whatever information is available. If you stop gathering information contradictory to what you believe, you do not have realistic beliefs. A belief is a temporary opinion that should grow until it becomes knowledge. If you gain knowledge contradicting your beliefs, change those beliefs. Knowledge helps you solve problems, whereas beliefs make problems worse. To solve a problem, you must suspend your beliefs.

Your beliefs are your own and should not come from others. You usually believe in what your parents believe when you are young. Over time, you may develop justifications for these beliefs, but your original beliefs were from other people. You do not brush your teeth because you believe in brushing your teeth. You brush your teeth because you know what will happen if you do not. We selectively gather beliefs and opinions from those we observe. The narrower the group we observe, the narrower our view of reality.

One problem with beliefs is anyone can believe anything. We do not require the beliefs to be factual. When you express something you believe to others, they must determine if you based what you are saying on reality. If the other person does not know better, they may take your statements as factual when you base them on opinions and biases. If you believe something based on unproven information or the beliefs of others, you are lying to everyone who you express your beliefs if you do not express them as beliefs.

Accepting your beliefs as untrustworthy is accepting the reality of your beliefs. Questioning your beliefs is crucial to turning your beliefs into knowledge. Scientists have a belief or hypothesis they test to prove their hypothesis true, false, or somewhere in between. Continuing to believe a hypothesis you or others have proven incorrect would be unscientific and illogical. Denying reality contradictory to your beliefs will handicap your life. Beliefs either correspond with reality or they deviate from it. The more your beliefs deviate from reality, the less you will accept it.

Depending on who you are talking to, you can change what you reveal about your beliefs. When you only selectively reveal your beliefs to certain people, it shows a lack of confidence in your beliefs. When I first discovered I was an atheist, I hid my atheism until I knew how others thought of religion. I believed God did not exist, just as they believed God existed. My belief was a judgment of other people, just as I worried they judged me. I eventually realized we were judging each other based on our own beliefs. When you accept reality, someone else's beliefs will not affect how you treat them.

Believing something does not make it real or unreal. Our beliefs come from not learning from our experiences, whereas our knowledge comes from learning from our experiences. We do not believe fire will burn us; we know fire will burn us. If you believe fire will not burn you, your beliefs are incorrect. We cannot prove most of our long-term beliefs to be correct or incorrect. Fire's effect on skin is simple knowledge. When you have a belief about a group of people, you declare your belief to be true about the entire group. If you knew something factual about every member, it would not be a belief. We can prove our beliefs real or unreal, but our beliefs are only a temporary step to gaining knowledge.

We base our future wants on hopes, dreams, and wishes we believe are possible. These wants are only helpful if we take steps to bring them to life. Many people hope for unrealistic things. We can hope for wings, but we know we will not have them in our lifetime. Merely hoping for something is not enough. If what you want is possible, you still need to act before it can happen. Wishing for a change will not change things. Hoping for something is the first step. Examining the reality of your dream and acting will make your wishes possible. What you hope for initially may change as you take steps toward it. This change is not abandoning your dreams; you are merely improving them.

Your beliefs should not control your actions or affect your behavior. Your beliefs can cloud your view of a situation. Fear, anxiety, and anger can develop from your beliefs. Your beliefs can cost you financially, emotionally, and in your relationships. People's beliefs create individual and societal problems. Because the beliefs are not visible, people blame their problems on the people and things they can see. People's beliefs separate them from other people and reality. Your actions should bring people closer to you, not separate you from them.

Removing people's long-term negative beliefs is necessary to help them accept reality. You must remove the beliefs carefully, so they do not view your attempts as an attack. Their beliefs are their reality. Helping them to accept realities that do not contradict their beliefs is a good starting place. You can eventually expand their view of reality to include their existing beliefs. They will only change their beliefs when they question them on their own. Be sure to point out the positive aspects of realities and avoid pointing out how their beliefs are destructive. Abandoning their beliefs can free them from the negativity their beliefs cause. The more they improve their life, the more they will accept additional realities.

Positive beliefs only reinforce what we know or think we know about the world. They do not change the world. Negative beliefs will pull you away from reality and impact your life negatively. Most negative emotions come from beliefs, and positive emotions come from reality. We should not attach emotions to our beliefs. People's attitudes come from their beliefs. Being positive or happy is not a belief. You do not believe you are happy; you are happy. If you believe you are happy, you may or may not be happy in reality. You can feel lonely even in a crowded room because of your negative beliefs. They create limits in your life, nurture self-fulfilling prophecies, and develop unhealthy thinking patterns. We blame our resulting misery on others, but our beliefs are truly to blame.

You will never accept all of reality until you remove your negative beliefs. Counting on a coincidence to develop into luck, a realized dream, or another belief we want to be true will not help you accomplish your goals. We should only hold beliefs until we can attain knowledge. Accepting reality is not about giving up on your dreams, it is about gaining the knowledge and skills to realize your dreams. The only belief helping you in this pursuit is believing in yourself.

Independent Thinking and Freewill

*"Freewill is an illusion. If you think
you control your actions, you're an idiot.
They have predestined everything we do to
happen long before any of us was here."*

Reality Denial

*"To say we don't have freewill just
seems like an excuse for people to do what
they want and blame it on others. If other
people pressured you to do things, you
accepted the pressure. If you don't like the
outcome, just accept you chose it and make
better decisions in the future."*

Reality Acceptance

Do we have freewill? Our brain is constantly multi-tasking regardless of our awareness of it. When you react to something, you are not consciously reacting to it, nor is something external helping you to react. Your brain is automatically reacting in your subconscious. Our thoughts work independently from other people's thoughts. If a group of people seems to think as one, they are merely syncing their behaviors with one another. Their minds remain independent. We can exercise freewill, but our beliefs allow us to deny the connection to our own thoughts. If your beliefs come from others, you feel even less freewill toward your actions. The more you understand reality, the more you can think independently.

Growing up, I was an extremely independent thinker. I knew my thinking differed from most other people. If everyone was doing something, that was the last thing I wanted to do. Standing out from others was much more important to me than fitting in. You might guess that I did not have a large group of friends and you would be right. My friends were independent thinkers like me. Weird conversations, actions, and thinking were our favorite activities. We were pointing out the absurdity of normal activities by questioning what is normal. Questioning your daily activities is an important part of life.

Much of our life is a mix of order and chaos. Our lives do not follow a predestined path. All the planning in the world cannot guarantee the future we desire. Anyone who claims to know the future is lying or playing the odds. Many things that have happened in the past will happen again. We should not confuse freewill with routine or a general cycle of the world. Most days have a beginning, middle, and end. A similarity between yesterday and today does not mean we have no choices in our daily lives.

A company can have a collective consciousness, but the individual people work independently to accomplish tasks as a group. There is usually one person who has more control over the group. A board of people may keep the person from harming the company or people in it, but the rest of the group is following the rules and orders from those above them. Individuals will follow the rules of the group rather than risk removal from it. People who break the rules know there will be consequences to their actions.

Everyone has freewill, but our fears and other emotions prevent us from behaving in random ways. Social norms tell us what we should do, but people can ignore them. What social norms you follow depends on what society you consider yours. We can split most societies into distinct cultures, groups, and structures. Some societies exercise more freewill than others. Some groups have more individually minded people, and others only see themselves as a part of a group. The more a society allows individual freedoms, the more the members will accept their own freewill. The more freewill you exercise in your life, the happier and healthier you will be.

SEE MORE EXAMPLES AT:

realityacceptance.com/category/thinking/independent-thinking/

realityacceptance.com/category/thinking/freewill/

Opinions

*"I have an opinion about everything.
If you tell me something is green, I have an
opinion about how green, whether it
should be green, and why green is not
real."*

Reality Denial

*"If I don't fully understand
something, I don't express an opinion
about it. I know that most of my opinions
are simply guesses about things I have
barely any knowledge of. An informed
opinion is the only one worth expressing."*

Reality Acceptance

You should not have an opinion about everything. If you do not understand something, you should not have an opinion about it. If you have not seen a movie, you should not express an opinion about it. We do not universally love or hate movies. The worst film and the best films will connect with some people and not connect with others. If you see a movie and you dislike it, you can express your opinion about it, but know others will disagree with you. Extremely positive or negative opinions mean less than a balanced opinion.

We express our opinions in actions, not words. If you express an opinion about something in words, you are investing a minimum amount of effort. If you force yourself to act, you are spending more time examining issues beyond a surface level reaction. Actions force you to be physically and mentally involved. If your opinion is we should observe all laws, show your opinion in your actions. Do not jaywalk, speed, liter, or break laws unless it is unsafe to do so. Talking to others who are breaking these laws will only push them away from listening to your opinions. As they say, actions speak louder than words.

Debates are examples of how useless conflicting opinions are at solving problems. When you can debate either side of an argument, your opinion means nothing. Politicians use these skills to express opinions about issues they know nothing about. These are skills they learned in the debates of their past. Calls to action and solutions were an integral part of the greatest speeches of all time. Actions and solutions are a minimal part of debates. Choosing a politician based on their actions and problem-solving skills is much better than choosing a politician by how well they debate with others. Much of the time, the winner of the debate is the best liar.

We give voters the responsibility of choosing who will represent us in the government. Whether the voting system works, the voters can express their opinion about their representatives. When people do not have an opinion about a vote and they still vote, their vote is a lie. There is no vote that is a win for all voters. We can hope for politicians who do their best for the most people, but few politicians fit this description.

My grandmother was someone who I would describe as brutally honest. A common story I tell about her (which makes it highly suspect) is when she asked my mom, "Do you think you'll ever replace these curtains?" With one question, my grandmother stated she did not like the curtains, thought my mom did not know how unattractive they were, and cared little for my mom's feelings. A promising idea is rarely the first thing that comes to your mind. If you do not recognize other people's feelings, your first thought will be a quick opinion based on a surface level view of the world. You do not need an opinion about everything.

Negative opinions do more harm than good. Opinions with words such as hate, stupid, ugly, or worse do not express an opinion as much as the negative state of the person expressing them. Negative critics of a piece of work express opinions of little use to others. Their reviews are often one-sided and long-winded opinions about what they did not like. Negative opinions are unhelpful and better left unexpressed.

People who do not deal with diverse points of view will eventually deny that any other point of view is valid. Without different opinions to make them think about their own, they will see their opinion as correct and factual. No opinion based on your beliefs is factual. They will see their opinions as the only reasonable ones. Dealing with diverse opinions will help you develop more well-rounded and positive opinions.

You can express your opinions quickly, but a logical opinion takes time. Taking the time to develop a logical opinion will yield a much more helpful opinion. If you do not know enough about something to express a logical opinion, invest the time to gather more information. We should base our opinions on our knowledge and experience with others relevant to the subject discussed. Take the time to see things from other points of view. Your opinion will be better and more logical the more information you consider.

Every sign of beauty depends on the opinions of others. Pursuing the mythical goal of beauty will always be subjective. The more diverse a group of people, the less they will agree on what is beautiful. Many factors go into what is beautiful to each person. Complete beauty is just as unattainable as perfection. People are not making themselves more beautiful when they put on make-up and other concealers of their flaws. They are disguising those flaws along with who they are as people. Being happy with yourself is the most beautiful expression you can show the world. People who are happy and healthy are beautiful.

SEE MORE EXAMPLES AT:

realityacceptance.com/category/thinking/opinions/

Reality Accepting Exercise:

Think about a problem in your life. Write only verifiable facts about the problem. Do not write what you believe about it. If you find yourself unable to state the problem fully, you can never solve it. Research anything you believe about it and turn your beliefs into knowledge. The more you learn about the problem, the more solutions you will find.

Chapter 13
Negative Thinking

*"If you have any brains at all, you'll
realize what a messed-up world this is and
give up. People who are happy got that
way by ignoring the negative people
around them. Their happiness disturbs
me."*

Reality Denial

*"Negative people think negatively. I
try to avoid them if I can. I definitely don't
ask them how they're doing. Negative
thinking leads to only seeing negativity in
the world. That doesn't sound like a fun
way to live life to me."*

Reality Acceptance

Negative thinking will never lead to a happy or healthy life.
When you think only negative thoughts, you will live a
negative and miserable life. People think negatively because
of their beliefs, experiences, and many other reasons. We learn
negative thinking from others, but continuing to think
negatively will lead you to teach others to think as you do. No
negative thoughts come from reality. Reality is not negative or
positive. You only accept aspects of reality you find negative,
but that is not accepting reality. You can only accept reality if
you get away from your negative thinking.

Negative thinking leads to negative behavior. When you
view the world through a negative lens, your negative

behavior becomes justifiable in your mind. You react with hostility to the world before the world can act hostile to you. Your hostile behavior seems logical to you as a reaction to the perceived hostility of others. Some of their hostile behavior is real, but to a much lesser extent than you are perceiving. Your negative beliefs justify your negative actions. Others may punish you for your hostile behavior while ignoring your negative thinking. Those punishing you may be blind to your inner turmoil because of their own inner conflicts. Focusing only on the hostile behavior will never address the negative thinking that is the true cause of your behavior.

The harmful effects of negative thinking remain invisible to many people. Others can tell you about your negative attitude, but you call yourself a realist. When someone else shows signs of negative thinking, you see them as negative because his negativity differs from yours. When you have health problems stemming from your negative thinking and behavior, you blame them on other factors not connected to the actual cause. Because other people are not in your head, they may accept your explanations.

You never consider your thinking when trying to find the cause of your health problems. As your health worsens, your health problems become more than just your negative thinking. Even improving your attitude is not enough to improve your health. Negative thinking will lead to mental and physical health problems. You blame your miserable life on a myriad of external problems when your negative thinking was the actual cause.

Ideologies

*"I believe my principles are sacred. If
we don't stand for something, we stand for
nothing. When people disagree with my
principles, they disagree with me. I will
fight them to the death!"*

Reality Denial

*"What I consider important in my life
changes all the time. How I see the world
changes the more diverse groups of people
I meet. A rigid system only benefiting how
a few people think does not work for
anyone."*

Reality Acceptance

An ideology is a rigid way of thinking. People develop a concept of the world that does not change, and they never question. The ideology of an individual or group confines thinking to a narrow spectrum of experiences and knowledge. They consider their beliefs equally with the knowledge they choose to accept. Any way of thinking based on beliefs rather than reality will lead to negative thinking and a degraded quality of life.

We originally conceived ideology as the science of ideas. Economic, political, and religious beliefs are the main things we have applied the term to since that time. We use it many times to condemn the negative policies of people and groups who see all other forms of thinking as misguided. When we only accept one way of thinking, we deny all other forms of thinking and reality with it. Choosing an ideology that does not change or grow leads to a culture which never advances beyond its simplistic origins. A culture that does not advance will always clash with other cultures that do. The culture that accepts reality will succeed far more than a culture that does not.

It is especially harmful when two ideologies conflict in a society. They will ignore any attempt to introduce actual issues into the dispute to prove the moral superiority of their ideology. Everyone on both sides of the conflict focuses on the competition of the ideologies while ignoring actual problems within the society. Social issues and concrete problems become worse because leaders are focusing on the ideological conflict. They may reach a decision on the superiority of the two ideologies while the society declines further into instability and reality denial.

SEE MORE EXAMPLES AT:

realityacceptance.com/category/thinking/ideologies/

Our Biases

*"I don't believe there is a bias toward
certain people in society over others.
White males are just more qualified for
most jobs. You may think I'm biased
because I'm a white male, but that's just
the way I see it."*

Reality Denial

*"I am constantly aware of my biases.
The best way to remain unbiased is to
research your decisions with as many
different people as you can. Diversity is
key to making any unbiased decision."*

Reality Acceptance

Bias comes from personal experience and beliefs. If you have
a personal connection with a subject or group, you will behave
favorably toward it. This can be conscious or subconscious,
but it draws you unequally to one choice over others. When
you look at something with preconceived notions, your beliefs
and emotions will shade your perceptions. Instead of seeing
the reality of it, you see a distorted view of it. The result of
biased thinking can lead to conflicts with others and a reduced
quality of life. It will force you to defend your unfair actions.
In reality, there is no defense.

Reality denial and bias gets worse with age. The more
you defend your biased practices, the better you will get at
maintaining them. This negative skill will pull you further
from your grasp of reality. Eventually, you will not remember
where your biases came from, and you will see them as the

most reasonable response. Accusations of bias will appear to you as prejudice from others, not you. When you fill your life with biased choices, you will find yourself alone.

When you are the recipient of a biased choice, you cannot accept the favorable treatment if you value reality. The adulation is unwarranted and accepting it will make you an accomplice to the biased crime. You have not earned the rewards you are receiving. Not considering all factors in what you accept about the world is not accepting reality. Ignorance is not an acceptable excuse for ignoring the biased choice. Your fear of losing the favorable treatment should not stop you from confronting the biased choice and pointing out the disparity. Accepting the reality of the situation may appear negative at first, but will eventually lead to a better outcome for everyone.

SEE MORE EXAMPLES AT:

realityacceptance.com/category/thinking/biases/

Reality Accepting Exercise:

Think about a reoccurring negative thought you have. It could be how much you hate your boss, hating your neighbor for disturbing you, hating how overweight you are, or simply hating Mondays. Are any of these thoughts a realistic assessment of the situation? Do they help you deal with the situation? Do you think other people do not know about your negative thoughts? Most of our negative thoughts lead to biases about ourselves or others. Negative thoughts come from negative beliefs. If you believe there is nothing you can do about something, your thoughts will grow more negative toward it. You can remove these negative thoughts by channeling your energy toward finding solutions to your problems. Many of the best solutions come from other people.

Chapter 14
Extreme Thinking

"I'm going to tell you something that is literally true. I'll die if everything doesn't go perfect tomorrow. If anything goes wrong, my life is over! If it goes perfectly, it will be the greatest day of my life."

Reality Denial

"Extreme people are hard to be around. Things are the greatest they've ever been or they're a disaster. They tire me out just being around them. If I ever find myself with an extreme opinion, I rethink it."

Reality Acceptance

Life is not a passing or failing grade. This all-or-nothing view of the world does not hold up to reality. Nothing is completely one extreme or another. When people think in extremes, they are attempting to simplify their view of the world. Extreme thinking leads to extreme emotions and extreme behavior. People who think this way can spiral into extreme actions that physically and psychologically damage themselves or others.

There are no winners and losers in life. Sports, games, politics, wars, and religion all claim to have winners and losers. In nature, the only winners are those who survive. Humans have developed well past those primitive days. Picking winners and losers based on arbitrary markers of success is a nod to those primitive times. Thinking of yourself as a winner or loser can lead to egotism or depression. People declaring themselves winners or losers are telling the world they are only capable of a simplistic and extreme view of themselves.

Nuance is the opposite of all-or-nothing thinking. When people only think in extremes, they ignore subtle details about the world and anything that is not extreme. This means they are missing most of life. Examining the minor deals of something allows you to glimpse the complexity of the world. Collecting these nuances of detail helps you build a more complete worldview. The more nuances you notice, the less extreme thinking you will do.

This or That Thinking

"You either get a job or you become a bum. I got a stressful job that I hate, but at least I'm not a bum. You want to see a bum? You should see my younger brother."

Reality Denial

"When people ask me to choose something with only two options, I ask for more options. Most of the time, the choices are so extreme from one another that my answer is none of the above. I have a long-time dislike of yes or no questions for this reason."

Reality Acceptance

Many people think there are only two choices in any decision. Very few decisions involve only two choices. They are attempting to simplify complex decisions. Sports, politics, religion, and schools have promoted the idea that there are winners or losers, good or bad people, and correct or incorrect answers. These are all examples of this or that thinking. Simple answers can only answer simple questions. Most realities involve complex questions that simple two choice thinking is inadequate to answer.

People get frustrated when they ask me a question with only two choices. I refuse to answer them because I point out there are many more than just two options for any question. They want me to answer it as I would a multiple-choice test. I have to point out to them I dislike multiple-choice tests because they oversimplify the choices. You can only answer simple questions with simple answers. Even simple questions require complex answers if you accept all the factors involved in reality. When people get to know me, they stop asking me simple two choice questions.

When people look for a cause-and-effect relationship, they are usually looking for a simple explanation of something. They want a single cause that leads to a single effect. There is rarely a single cause or effect of anything. There may be major causes and effects emerging from the rest, but smaller factors can contribute to the result. Scientists in the lab can create simple cause-and-effect relationships, but life in the actual world is more complex. When talking about historical events, people try to simplify them into cause-and-effect relationships. Every person who is a part of the historical event contributes distinct factors to the cause and effect. Singling all those factors down to a few causes and effects is impossible.

As with all extreme thinking, this or that thinking is an attempt to simplify life into extremes. Only by ignoring most of reality can we find this thinking convincing. Simple answers and simple questions do not address most of reality. To simplify the complexity of the world is to ignore the reality of the world. People dislike unknowable questions and complex answers. We do not need a full understanding of the world to accept reality. Understanding reality will lead us to the best possibilities for understanding what we can know about the world.

Disasters and Tragedies

*"I do not handle disasters well. Last
year when I lost my job, I was
inconsolable. My life was in ruins. I
couldn't do anything. I'm in a job now, but
I live in fear it will end tragically."*

Reality Denial

*"Whenever a disaster or tragedy
happens, people usually turn to me. I
handle most situations with calm logic. I
handle major problems such as floods or
earthquakes like any other problem. My
primary concerns are making sure people
are okay and safe. That includes myself
because I can't help others if I'm injured.
Then we work on damage to things."*

Reality Acceptance

Disasters and tragedies force reality on everyone involved in
them. They force you to confront realities you may have tried
to ignore or deny in the past. Some people see disasters where
none exist. You may feel it is a tragedy if you lose your job,
but it is merely a problem you need to solve. True disasters
and tragedies are complex problems we cannot solve easily.
They involve many factors happening concurrently, resulting
in an unknowable future for a group or community of people.
It is at these times when extreme thinking does not help.

Most people are at their best in a disaster. Petty daily
concerns do not have time to enter their thoughts. We come
together to accept the reality of these tragic events. We help

one another and work as a community to solve the most pressing problems as they come up. Some people will respond to the disaster badly, but most people accept the responsibility their actions can have in the community. If you think in extremes before the disaster, you will continue this extreme thinking during a disaster. Disasters force most people into accepting reality, but not all.

Offering prayers for victims of a tragedy or disaster only helps the person offering the prayers. We can only help the victims by actions to keep them safe and helping them solve problems. Knowing you are thinking about the victims may give them some comfort, but you are not taking actions to help their situation. The tragedy confirms the beliefs most religions hold; everything happens for a reason. This simple thinking denies the reality of what we need during a tragedy. Helping others with our actions, money, and empathy is what they need most.

Extreme thinkers use tragedies as proof of the downfall of humanity. Religious leaders declare a tragedy as punishment for a group of sinners. Other people use tragedies as an excuse to give up on the world. Your life after a tragedy will definitely change, but it is not over. The tragedy is a wake-up call that nothing in life is permanent. You may have lost fundamental parts of your life. We can replace physical items. Many people are willing and able to help you replace them. Human lives are not replaceable.

Disasters and tragedies are having fewer devastating effects on people's lives than they did in the past. Extreme thinkers exaggerate the devastation well beyond the reality of the situation. They allow their beliefs to ignore or deny what others accept. This may be difficult to keep in mind when you are in the middle of a tragic event, but it is the reality of the situation. Accepting this reality will allow you to solve the problems caused by the disaster or tragedy sooner.

SEE MORE EXAMPLES AT:

realityacceptance.com/category/thinking/disasters-and-tragedies/

The News Media

Reality Denial

Reality Acceptance

The news media of today has changed drastically from its origins. We disseminated the news first in print. They delivered much of the news to the public who had no other way of getting it. It was a democratizing process, allowing the dissemination of information relevant to people's lives. The reality of people in power, governmental policies, and institutional corruption could no longer remain hidden from the public. The news could be independent, transparent, ethical, and serve the public interest. Unfortunately, this idyllic vision of the news no longer exists.

Today's news media no longer has a monopoly on public information. The multitude of outlets include print media, video and audio news, and the enormous selection of news sites online. In any one category, several outlets are competing to get you to read, watch, or listen to their news over other outlets. Their priority is no longer to inform the public about news relevant to them, but to gather information that will keep people reading, watching, or listening to their version of events. They are informing the public of irrelevant information that will keep people interested long enough to present ads to them.

Because positive news is not as highly rated, most news stories are negative. We call them news stories because most of them are stories meant to entertain. I do not find most negative entertainment interesting, but many people do. The news presents stories to invoke fear, anxiety, sadness, and anger because emotions are the easiest way to get people interested. The more people watch the news, the more emotional they get, and the more they continue to watch more news. People can become addicted to watching the news just as they get addicted to binge watching a television series. The news is their form of entertainment, from which they only attain a surface level of understanding of any subject.

We might consider it harmless to entertain ourselves with the news, but it is a negative and unrealistic form of entertainment that claims to represent reality. When we view the negative and hateful depictions of the world, it is negative and harmful to our thinking. I do not watch the news for the same reason I do not watch most horror films. Feeling afraid and anxious is not entertaining for me. What makes one disaster better or worse than another is the sensational manner in which they present them. You come away from most stories feeling worse than if you did not watch the news.

Car chases are an extreme form of the negativity found in television news. They are unhealthy for the people in the chases and the people who watch them. People driving from the police are trying to escape the reality of their situation. Fear clouds their perception. No rational person sees a car chase as a logical decision by the driver. The news represents the car chase as a race through city streets and highways with capture or escape as the two outcomes. In reality, the people driving never gets away, and they injure many people with their actions. The news sensationalizes their behavior for ratings. It is no longer news for the public good.

The news must present biased accounts of events to cater to their audience. This biased accounting is political, social, religious, or presenting other biases of their audience. We have added an extra layer of bias to the news in the form of advertisers. They must not only please their audience, but their advertisers. They have no choice but to agree to any demands the advertiser has about stories, especially if they involve the advertiser. The news has removed the former independence, transparency, ethics, and serving of the public from its origins. It leaves us with a negative form of entertainment that misleads rather than informs.

Reality Accepting Exercise:

Think of someone you know who always handles problem situations without freaking out. Now think of someone you know who handles all situations, no matter how small, by automatically freaking out. What are the differences between these people? Does freaking out help the situation? Do you want to be around someone freaking out during a situation? Unfortunately, the differences that allow them to freak out or not are all in their heads. The only outside sign of how they think is in their actions. How they think about situations changes how they deal with them. If you freak out in situations, think about all the things you fear will happen. How likely are they to happen? Are there usually other people around who can help you? Think about what could realistically happen and write several solutions for each of them. When you are in this situation in the future, think about this list. Refine the list over time as different versions of the situation come up. Your anxiety level will improve over time, and you will freak out less.

SEE MORE EXAMPLES AT:

realityacceptance.com/category/thinking/the-news-media/

Chapter 15
Competitive Thinking

"Life is a competition that I plan on winning. I am competitive about everything I do. When I play a game, I play to win. Other people say it's no fun playing with me, but those people are losers."

Reality Denial

"I would much rather cooperate with other people than compete with them. Playing games on the playground was fun. When I got older and most of the other players cared about winning, it just wasn't fun anymore."

Reality Acceptance

Competition has existed in the world since creatures competed for resources, space, and sexual partners. Humans today think mainly of the competitions existing in sports, politics, education, business, and society. These are artificial versions of natural ones. We no longer compete for resources, space, and sexual partners directly. We perpetuate a myth that life is a competition. This competitive thinking has led to a distorted view of life which devalues humanity's connections to one another.

Competition only works positively for society with cooperation. We must cooperate to distribute a few resources to an overpopulated world. This requires us all to cooperate and compromise our wants and needs. If we do not, we further separate ourselves from one another. This leads to societies that argue, fight, and go to war to avoid having to compromise. Our competitive thinking allows us to live unhappy and unhealthy lives because winning is all that matters. It pleases us when we win, but that pleasure does not last. The competition shifts up a level as we compete with others who have also won. It forces us to cooperate with others, but the end goal is raising ourselves above them. When you raise yourself to the top level, you find yourself alone.

The main global competition that we have today is in economics. We are no longer exchanging goods and services for other goods and services. We have created a monetary system to access our value as people. The more money you have, the more powerful you can become. The more powerful you become, the more money you can get. We deprive many people of basic life necessities while a few people live in wasteful overabundance. Religions have declared the love of money the root of all evil while holding services in wastefully overabundant churches. Money is not the problem. We would not have hospitals, schools, or homes without it. The problem is in treating money as a competition. Again, competition without cooperation is negative for society.

Most people count their steps so they can point out to others how many more steps they took than them. They do not care about the health benefits as much as raising their score relative to other people. Anything you add competition to will devalue it.

- Help + competition = judgment.
- Money + competition = business.

- Play + competition = games.
- Exercise + competition = sports.
- Happiness + competition = pride.
- Entertainment + competition = simple art.

If you find nothing wrong with the outcome of adding competition to these things, you are a competitive thinker. Hopefully, you realize the destructive nature of this thinking before it affects your health. The major health problem from competitive thinking is stress. The major cost to society is separating us from one another.

SEE MORE EXAMPLES AT:

realityacceptance.com/category/thinking/competitive-thinking/

Reality Accepting Exercise:

Think of an activity you enjoy that involves competition. Write about all the things you enjoy about it. Do you enjoy getting together with other people? Does it take place in a location you enjoy? Does the activity involve physical activities and exercise? Are you able to learn new skills each time you do the activity? Look at the list and note how many of the things you enjoy require competition. If you enjoy the competitive parts of an activity, do you still enjoy them if you lose the competition? You probably skipped this exercise or even this entire chapter if you are a competitive thinker. If you are not, I would encourage you to think about the parts of a competition you enjoy and do those without the competitive parts.

Chapter 16
What Should Be

"The government should take the same amount of taxes from everyone. There should be no loopholes available to anyone. If I was in charge of the government, I would quit doing things that don't make any sense."

Reality Denial

"What should be is not what is. The moment people talk about how things should be, you know that is not how they are. Saying what should be is not the hard part. The hard part is getting what should be to become a reality. Saying what should be is much easier than getting things to change."

Reality Acceptance

What you think should be is rarely the reality of a situation. It has less to do with the ethics of the world than your satisfaction with your life. Everyone's opinions about what should be the reality will differ. Your ability to change a situation or problem depends on your ability to connect with others. If you have power, you can order others to implement your wishes, but most people will disagree with your decision. If you can connect with others and explain your plan to them, they will agree with your decision more.

We should never compare ourselves to other people. The things we like about their lives are based on an outward view of them. We control all our senses and actions with our brains. It takes years to get to know others, and we can still never truly know how they perceive the world. Most of us barely understand how our own minds work. If we did, we would know that comparing ourselves to others is a waste of time and energy.

Trying to understand other people's minds is impossible. If you admire how someone else handles life, ask them about how they think and view the world. How someone thinks is who they are as a person. Changing how you think will change your life. Positive thinking will lead to positive outcomes in your life. Worrying about what should be will lead to believing you have no control of your life. Achieving what should be is a matter of realistically examining what could be and working to make it what is.

SEE MORE EXAMPLES AT:

realityacceptance.com/category/thinking/what-should-be/

Logical Ethics

*"I try to do the right thing, but
sometimes the right thing is not exactly
legal. If I'm taking my child to the
hospital, I'm going to break every law to
get her there. Other drivers need to
understand that my child comes first."*

Reality Denial

*"If something makes little sense
ethically, it is not logical. If I do something
that only works for me, it is neither logical
nor ethical. Logic does not work unless it
considers all factors involved in
something. A decision is not logical if it
does not work ethically for everyone."*

Reality Acceptance

The ethical choice is the most logical choice when considering
all available information. When you only consider an issue
from a narrow perspective, you will often reach the most
unethical and illogical conclusion. If you mismatch your ethics
with the rest of society, you will not agree logically with the
rest of society. Logic and ethics do not exist in a bubble. Your
personal ethics must be as flexible as your societal logic.

When I have made questionable ethical choices, I usually
focus on a singular goal guiding my decisions. If I am
weaving in and out of traffic and cutting people off, I focus
more on being late than on making logical driving decisions.
Both logic and ethics consider safety, empathy, efficiency, and
health. I drive safely so other vehicles can be safe and I can

get to work without stress or injuries. My driving is logical only if it is ethical.

Doing the right thing can be difficult when it conflicts with other rules in your life. A sign can read "stay off the grass," but you ignore it if your two-year-old is walking into a hole in the grass. Logic dictates breaking the rule is the ethical thing to do. If someone is driving in the wrong lane and they head straight toward you, your adherence to the law is at your own risk. Rules, just like the lines on the road, are guides for your behavior. They establish guidelines, but you will not automatically add them to the programming of your brain. You must know when to adhere to them and when it is logical to ignore them.

When people view logic and morality as different, it is often because of their beliefs. Without a moral rule forbidding murder, they cannot deduce that murder is illogical. They can, but they do not see killing someone as a logical and moral choice. They believe without rules there is chaos. In reality, every other species except humans operates without written or verbal rules to guide them. All they have is their inner logic. If it is logical to kill one of their own kind for the good of their species, it is the ethical choice. Murder is not inherently unethical. Ethics, especially with murder, are complex and we can only learn them through experience and practice with logical thinking.

Many people think of logic and reason as a ridged set of rules that will lead to one logical outcome. The more factors involved in a logical decision; the more outcomes are probable. If you only consider a few factors, you are deciding with little information on what you believe is correct. People go to prison based on these illogical decisions. We punish them because of their immoral behavior, but we would have better results teaching them the skills of logical thinking. The older we get, the more logical and ethical our decisions become.

Just because you can do something does not mean you should. Most people know this, but some people do not fully understand the difference between what they can and should do. They do not have logical thinking skills. A kid will say, "Well, you didn't tell me I couldn't hit my sister." His parents can tell him it is not right to hit others. They make it a moral issue. This does not explain why it is illogical to hit others. You can take him through the steps of logical thinking. What did he hope to gain from his actions? Is he angry at his sister? Is he lashing out because he is jealous of his sister? Like any lesson, it will take time for him to learn, but he will be more prepared for life if he learns logical thinking skills.

SEE MORE EXAMPLES AT:

realityacceptance.com/category/thinking/logical-ethics/

Regrets

> *"I have many regrets in my life. I
> wish I didn't drink so much, take so many
> drugs, treat my kids so badly, let my
> diabetes get out of control, and handle all
> of my relationships so horribly. The car I
> fixed up in high school is still in my
> possession. It's the one thing I don't regret
> keeping."*
>
> Reality Denial

> *"When I make big life decisions, I
> think about what decision I would regret
> the least. Avoiding regrets is the best way
> to live your life. I will always regret
> decisions I made based on fear or anger."*
>
> Reality Acceptance

We all have regrets in our lives. We regret the things we said, the things we did, and how we lived our lives. These regrets affcct our health and happiness, but do not change reality. Recognizing these regrets for what they are is important to dealing with them. They are all poor decisions from our past that we wish we could live over. Learning from our poor decisions will help us make better decisions in the future. Once we recognize this, we can prevent ourselves from having regrets at the end of our lives.

The best way to avoid regrets is learning from your failures. If you focus only on your regretful behavior, you will not learn from that behavior. Instead of focusing on what you should have done, focus on how you thought during a situation. Most times, our emotions guide us in a regretful situation. Denying your emotions will only make things worse. Instead, examine why you were in that emotional state. Examine the triggers for your emotions and avoid them.

Regretful events are mainly about what lead to them. If others were behaving badly, ignore their behavior in your reexamining of events. The only person you can control is yourself. We do not logically think out regretful situations in our minds. They happen from negative emotions and thoughts that cloud our logical thinking. If you yell at your co-workers, it is not about them. It is about how you feel about your working conditions. The emotional outburst shows your inner turmoil. Most times, an examination of your emotions will lead to the explanation of the regretful event.

When you identify the genuine sources of regrets, you must implement changes to learn from them. The necessary changes may be internal, external, or a combination. If you continue to have regretful events at work, your work life needs to change. You may need to get a new job, change your work environment, or discuss your concerns with coworkers or a supervisor. This will change your routine and take some adjustments for you, but is vital to preventing future regrets. To change a situation, you must examine it and understand where the problems are.

There are many regrets we wait to the end of our lives to confront. The best way to live life is to avoid these regrets. If parts of your daily life are making you unhappy or unhealthy, you will regret these things if you do not change them. These regrets are symptoms of how you think. Negative thinking will cause more regrets at the end of your life. Avoid these regrets by eliminating the sources of your negative thinking throughout your life.

SEE MORE EXAMPLES AT:

realityacceptance.com/category/thinking/regrets/

Reality Accepting Exercise:

Think about something you think other people should do differently. How much do you know about why they do it the way they do? Is the way you would do it completely different from the way they do it? Have you tried doing it the way they do it? If so, what did you find incorrect about their way of doing it? What are the advantages of the way you do it or would do it? Is it quicker, require less energy, safer, more efficient, or better in some other way?

Now think about the advantages of your way. Would other people see them as advantages? Do you think you value the same things as other people? Because we can do something faster or more efficiently does not make it better for everyone. We often judge others without knowing their true motivations for their actions. Sometimes people do things a certain way because that is how they have always done them. They may not even remember why they do it that way. If they seem receptive, can ask them why they do it that way, and make suggestions. They may surprise you and point out an advantage to their method you did not think about.

Chapter 17
Fear of the Unknown

"I don't like things that don't have clear-cut answers. Meeting new people, going someplace new, or being in a situation I've never been in are things I avoid. I don't know how to act in unfamiliar situations. You can keep your new experiences to yourself."

Reality Denial

"New experiences excite me. I love meeting new people and going to unknown places. Learning new things about the world makes life interesting."

Reality Acceptance

One of my favorite words is ambiguity. Most people fear ambiguity. It is a fear of the unknown. This can be a problem because life has few straightforward answers. I find ambiguity exciting. Things are more interesting when I do not understand them easily. When you enter an unknown situation, the possibilities are endless. Few new situations turn out as badly as we think they will. Most of the time, they turn out much better than we expect.

People fear the unknown because they believe the fears in their brain will come true. The only place your nightmares come true is in your dreams. Reality is far less dramatic. Planning for disasters that never happen means you will see disasters everywhere. Dealing with your fears is about dealing with your thinking. The only fear you do not have control of is someone or something startling you suddenly. The things you fear about the unknown are mostly in your mind.

Focus on the positive possibilities of a situation when confronted with something new. Meeting someone new could result in finding your new best friend. Navigating a fresh path could lead to a better and more satisfying route for your life. These possibilities are much more likely than any fears you have constructed in your mind. When you look for positive possibilities, you will find them everywhere.

Time is arbitrary, but that is fine. Humans created the concept of time to organize our lives. No other species observes a concept of time except the ones dictated by nature. We have clocks on our wrists, on our walls, in our vehicles, and in our computers. Our technology has become dependent on the accuracy of time. We tell ourselves we depend on time, but it is not true. Our dependence on time is as arbitrary as time itself.

It throws our sense of timing off if we do not have an accurate time to reference. We depend on sources of time to tell us when to get up, when to work, and when we have time to do nothing. Planning our day means scheduling our time. None of this happens in other species. Humans do not live natural lives. This does not mean we cannot get back to a more natural way of living. It also does not mean we have to abandon our concept of time all together. The key is balance.

Balancing your dependence on time means only observing time when it is necessary. We cannot completely abandon our dependence on time. You could not live in the modern world without it. Knowing when to observe time is a skill you will need to develop. If you constantly refer to time throughout your day, this is a habit you need to break. If you do not breathe, you could die. The same is not true for observing time.

SEE MORE EXAMPLES AT:

realityacceptance.com/category/thinking/fear-of-the-unknown/

realityacceptance.com/category/thinking/ambiguity/

Change

Reality Denial

Reality Acceptance

Change is important to growing and learning as a person. Your first day of school is a change that can lead to developing who you will become. We all fear change to varying degrees. Change happens all the time. Most of it, we do not notice. If it is a change affecting our lives, we notice it. We can deny it, but it is now a reality. Accepting change is just as important as accepting reality. Change is a constant part of our lives, but without it, our lives would be dull.

Not accepting change will lead to more change. If you do not accept one change, other changes will build out of control because you cannot control what you do not accept. Your denial will grow until you reject most realities you found unacceptable. People spend many hours complaining about change when dealing with it would be a better use of their time. Words do not affect change; actions do.

Negative changes in your life are problems in need of solutions. Minor changes may never affect your life. Major changes definitely will. Many people view change as a tragedy, but these changes are only events which will require a fresh way of thinking about a situation. Each change you deal with leads to increasing your problem-solving skill. The more changes you handle successfully, the more confidence you will develop for handling future changes.

Planning for change will help you deal with change. Denying or ignoring change does not work, but expecting and planning for it will. Not expecting change is like not expecting reality. You can plan for change regardless of the change. Signs of future change are all around us. Clouds in the sky may show a change in the weather. When people find themselves unaware of a change that has already happened, they ignore the signs of it. Paying attention to the world around you is the best way to see change coming. Accepting it is the first step to dealing with it.

Reality Accepting Exercise:

Think about a time in your life when you went through a dramatic change. You could have moved, lost a job, got married, went to a new school, had a serious accident, or had some other uncontrollable change happen. Do you remember planning for the change? Did you expect it to go well? Were you thinking that the change would ruin your life? Did it ruin your life? Were other people affected by the change positively or negatively? When you think about the change, did it help you grow as a person?

Change is never completely positive or negative. If nothing ever changed in your life, it would become monotonous. How you view the change shows how it will affect you. Speculating about the change is not as important as planning for it. If you plan on freaking out from the change, you will. Your only job during a change is to prevent future problems. You can view change as exciting or frightening, but the change is the same.

Chapter 18
Religious Thinking

"Thank God the doctor could save me. It's a miracle I didn't die when my heart stopped. God answered all my prayers by saving my life. Praise the lord!"

Reality Denial

"I find devout religious people hard to talk to. They have such a narrow view of the world. I see the diverse wonder and beauty of our complex world and they reduce it all to supernatural beings controlling it all. The reality of the world is much more interesting."

Reality Acceptance

In this chapter, I will talk about religious thinking. You can skip this chapter if you have accepted the other realities I present in this book, but do not want to hear my thoughts on religion. I am not religious myself, so my thoughts are as an outsider. In reading books on reality, happiness, and health, I found many of them contained spiritual practices unhelpful to attaining the major goals of the books. I have also read books on atheism, but they were mostly negative attacks on religion, unhelpful for accepting other realities outside of religion. I will not insult or compliment religion, but I see belief as an inadequate tool for examining reality. Having said that, I say goodbye or welcome.

We cannot agree on a definition of what makes up a religion, but I will attempt one for religious thinking. We could define religious thinking as the collective supernatural beliefs of a group of people who cannot prove whose beliefs. When people disagree on the collective beliefs, they start a new religion or join a religion more suited to their beliefs. We do not require religion to be a member of some societies while it is mandatory in others. If you are religious, you are just as capable of accepting reality as a non-religious person unless it comes to your religious beliefs.

I took a Science Fiction as Literature course in the early years of attending college. The instructor of the class told me I would wind up being a Buddhist. He knew I was an atheist and was an atheist himself before he studied Buddhism. Buddhism is a mix of spirituality and a realistic view of life. He was right that I disliked religions that openly ignored reality, but he was wrong that I would embrace the spirituality of Buddhism. Because a religion views spirituality as positive does not make spirituality real. From a scientific point of view, there is no evidence for anything beyond the brain creating movement in living beings. Without a brain, the only thing a living organism can do is grow toward other things. Scientists who are also religious have searched for evidence of spirits and have come up empty.

Most religions do not accept the finite nature of life. From concepts such as the afterlife, eternity, and infinite power, religious leaders tell their followers about the infinite possibilities available in the religion. When your body and brain die, you can live on in the afterlife for eternity and experience the infinite power of a higher being. There are no limits to the amount of pleasure or pain anyone can feel.

Limitless possibilities are fortunately not possible because limitless possibilities for one person means limited possibilities for other people.

If any one thing in life was limitless, it would limit everything else. The finite nature of life allows the diversity of life we see. If dinosaurs did not die out, humans would not be a dominant species. The ability of humans to adapt, deal with limited resources, and overcome diversity has allowed us to survive despite these limitations. To hold on to the belief that supernatural beings predestined you to thrive only discounts our contributions to our own existence. These limits allow us to live longer, happier, and healthier lives. A limitless life would be a downgrade.

We have used religion to advance societies, but also to degrade them. Before science existed, religion answered people's questions about the world. It gave them concrete answers to complex questions. This is where religion diverts from science. We can only answer complex questions with complex answers. To attain these answers, we must examine every aspect of reality and prove our assertions. I found in authoring this book investigating reality involves several factors I can only touch on. The more proof of something being real, the more we accept it in science. Religion requires faith and only offers unverifiable anecdotes as proof.

One person's belief is another's disbelief. I accept the people who follow religions, though I do not accept their religions. I understand why people believe in religions, but I will never believe in one myself. We do not have to believe in reality for it to exist. Understanding reality requires accepting what we can know about it. The more I learn about reality, the more excited I get to continue my investigation of it. The things I discover rarely disappoint me. Trying to advance my knowledge of reality gets me out of bed in the morning.

Religions explain their supernatural beliefs partly in fables and allegories. Many of the stories contain lessons on how to live your life. You can learn the same lessons from secular fiction without the claims of the stories being true. I find secular fiction more interesting to read because they focus on the reality of people's lives. The stories focus mostly on people dealing with life without accepting reality. If characters accept reality, they are usually the hero. We do not mark religious stories as fiction because people believe in them, not because they base them on reality.

I am in favor of supernatural things existing, but I know they do not. It would be great if dragons, ghosts, and fairies existed, but there is no evidence they do. I am definitely not in favor of gods existing. The concept of gods is antithetical to a concept of freewill. If we act as predestined people, our choices are not our own. Creating a purpose for my life keeps me excited about the future. Thinking of myself as the puppet of a supernatural being makes me feel as if I am living in a horror film. I do not enjoy most horror films, and I do not want to live in one.

Religions are an attempt to simplify our perceptions of life. They present simplified rules for living with answers people can easily believe and follow. These beliefs only affect their lives positively inside the religion. If someone only learns about reality from their religion, they will be incapable of handling non-religious problems. The first step in handling any problem is understanding the reality of the problem. None of the simplified religious rules work to solve actual problems.

Many people believe in a religion with no real understanding of all aspects of it. They understand the ceremonies, traditions, and their place in it, but do not look beyond this basic knowledge. People can only believe in a religion if they think it is improving their lives. They accept the religion regardless of their understanding of it. Religion only requires knowledge of enough of the religion to follow its rules. Faith is an easy requirement of followers, but religious knowledge is unnecessary and difficult to attain.

Discovering something you did not know existed is not a miracle. Getting help when you need it is realizing there has been help for you all along. You did not see the help before because you did not need it. Thanking the people who help you is much more important than thanking a supernatural being. Accepting the reality of who helped you is accepting reality. Religious thinking clouds people's views of reality, so they ignore the genuine source of the help they receive. They only accept the reality that lines up with their religious views. Religion does not help you accept reality, but it does not have to prevent you from accepting it.

The Religious Elephant in the Room

People turn to their religion in times of turmoil. When they do not know what to do in their life, they turn to a higher power to guide them. They believe they are incapable of deciding on their own and do not recognize or know about the real help around them. To realize we are all on earth with no direction other than the one we create for ourselves is a scary thought for some people. Most people search for a purpose in life, but some people want their purpose imparted to them. The less involved you are in creating your purpose, the less the purpose is yours.

Why would you leave a religion that provides for your family, helps raise your kids, and tells you about your true potential? The only thing the religion requires of you is your faith. These would all be positive things if they were true. Religion requires donations, will not buy a house for you, will not send your kids to college, and is lying to you about your potential unless it is supplying you with concrete ways to change your life for the better. Telling you anything is possible is not an encouragement, it is a lie.

We must accept unquestionable truths on faith because they are not actual truths. If they were real, they could withstand any amount of questioning. When we are kids, we ask our parents if we should do certain things. Some parents answer these questions to the best of their knowledge. Other parents say the tried-and-true, "Because I said so." My favorite question when I was a kid was, "Why?" To this day, I cannot accept doing something without knowing why I am doing it. Religion will never work for me because I question everything.

A dog has a much simpler mind than a human. If you yell at a dog to stop doing something, he or she will usually stop doing it. Human brains are much more highly developed. Being skeptical of things helps guide us. It has prevented us from many dangerous situations. Fear is healthy for our wellbeing, but knowledge can help us deal with the fear. When we have blind faith in something, we bypass our fears and ignore dangerous realities. We may also ignore realities that could help us. Religion can be dangerous if it allows you to ignore reality.

The fear of society not accepting us, our parents, or our friends is why people join or stay with a religion. If everyone in your life is religious, you cannot imagine life without it. Life outside of religion seems chaotic to you. Alongside the unknown factors of a secular life, you know negative reactions from your family and friends are inevitable. If your beliefs are not harming others and you are happy and healthy most of the time, there is no reason for you to change. Judging your life from your closed off view may hide the reality of your life. Without viewing your life outside of the religion, you may miss your best life.

It will be difficult to remove the filters of your beliefs, but necessary to take control of your life. If you claim to be happy while experiencing an above average amount of anger, anxiety, fear, or sadness, you are lying to yourself. These behaviors are outward signs of inner turmoil. Find time to have positive experiences outside of your religion. These experiences should help you avoid your negative emotions and not involve your beliefs. If you find yourself able to sustain positive emotions, your beliefs have caused your negative emotions.

Translating Religion into Reality Acceptance

Religion has many positive aspects that accept reality and connect people socially. The supernatural elements of religion deny much of reality and take your focus away from important elements of your life. You can accept the positive elements of religion without accepting the negative. The supernatural side of religion leads to beliefs about reality that are negative and harmful to the followers. You do not have to be a member of a religion to learn from the religion. We can translate most of the beliefs coming from religion into Reality Acceptance.

Removing yourself from religious beliefs will involve replacing former beliefs with fresh ways of thinking based on an acceptance of reality. Old habits and routines will change, but only after you have changed your thinking. Beliefs you held for years will take time to replace. Establishing fresh ways of thinking will also take time. Changing your life in one day should not be your goal. Your goal in the beginning is to accept new realities every day.

Changing your social connections from your religion can be the most troublesome part of accepting reality. This may include your family, friends, or the people you only know through your religion. The good news is you need not replace any of them. You are changing your thinking about the religion, not your entire social network. Thinking differently to other people does not mean you cannot interact with them. If you did not interact with friends or family who thought differently to you, this may seem difficult. Allow yourself time to notice the reality in your life before you make behavioral changes.

Following is a set of realistic and positive replacements for religious beliefs:

- You can replace the **higher power** you believe in with reality. In reality, we trust. Praise be to reality. Reality is good. Reality will not judge you, does not require worship, is everywhere, and will always provide you with solutions to your problems. As with any higher power, you must actively seek the truth from reality.

Instead of praying for answers, you can accept the reality of existing answers.

- **Faith** in religion is unquestionable. You can have a faith in reality that you can always question. The more you know about reality, the more you will view the world positively. It will not present you with clear and simple answers, but realistic information. You can test your faith in reality, but you will strengthen it the more you know about it.

- Your **spirit or soul** is the accumulation of your memories, emotions, and personality. It lives in your brain with your other thoughts. We want to see the spirits of other people because they represent our memories of them. If they are positive memories, we see them as good spirits. If they are negative memories, we see them as evil spirits. Ghosts do not exist, but your memories do.

- **Evil** does not exist, but extremely negative people do. What people call evil is a denial of realities you accept. They believe their actions are just as you believe they are evil. Evil implies they do not have control of their actions. The devil does not possess them; their extremely negative emotions and beliefs guide their actions.

Reality Accepting Exercise:

Think about your views on religion. Are you religious, non-religious, or somewhere in between? Now think about someone you know who is extremely religious and someone you know who is extremely non-religious. If you do not know anyone personally who is extreme, think of a celebrity who fits the profile. Can you see these two extremes having a constructive conversation about religion? Are there things they would agree on? Would you be able to moderate the conversation and find things they could both agree on? Could you state each of their point of views without bias or inserting your own opinion?

Religion is a belief system that does not require having the same belief system to understand. People's religious beliefs are as varied and different as non-believers'. Someone from the same religion can have differing views about the religion and the world. How we view religion differs from how we view the world. If people are from a certain religion, you do not see their beliefs in their actions. You only see their actions. We should only judge others by their actions, not their beliefs.

Part 5
Behavior

Chapter 19

The Reality of Your Behavior

"My parents, teachers, and bosses always said I had behavior problems. The only problem was them all taking my behavior seriously. My behavior is entertaining to people who like good practical jokes. Hardly anyone has gotten hurt by me, and only a few people cried."

Reality Denial

"I behave differently when I'm around different people. Know your audience. Especially around people you don't know you need to take cues from their behavior. I am always aware of how my behavior affects everyone around me."

Reality Acceptance

People view the behavior of others as a sign of who they are as people. Our behaviors result from our beliefs, emotions, and experiences from the past. Behavior is the physical manifestation of our mental health. We judge others by their behavior, but we know our own behavior is not always who we are inside. Examining the behaviors of other people shows who they are most of the time. We have to piece together their behaviors as clues to their mental state.

I grew up with an inability to ignore others. My sensory overload problems made me abundantly aware of my effect on others. This ensured my behavior was appropriate most of the time and increased my awareness of what behavior was appropriate. As an adult, I understand the motivations for people's behaviors better than most people do. Our emotions have more to do with our behavior than the behavior of others. Behaving inappropriately stems from emotional problems. If we ignore or deny our emotional problems, our inappropriate behavior will continue.

Understanding the behavior of others requires understanding our own behavior. A single behavior is not enough to judge them by. If we have a series of strange behaviors throughout our day, people who know us can piece together explanations for our behavior. Strangers can behave differently, but we would not know it. Putting yourself in their shoes will help, but we will never understand others by their behavior alone.

Judging the behavior of others requires examining multiple behaviors. If you are not aware of your own behavior, you cannot judge the behavior of others. Translating their behavior into an evaluation of them as people takes skill and is never fully accurate. You must consider the time, place, and circumstances of their behavior. Your experiences, knowledge, and understanding of human nature will influence the factors you consider. Quick judgments will only lead to misunderstandings.

The amount of reality you accept will affect your behavior. It will influence your health, beliefs, thinking, and relationships with others. Our behavior stems from all these things, but it can also influence them. Poor health can lead to denying science. This can cause denial of other realities. Denying reality can lead to a belief that your behavior does not affect others. Your behavior affects everyone you interact with. Believing differently denies the reality that other people exist.

Repeated behaviors will eventually become habits. Negative habits will lead to more negative habits. A lifetime of negative habits will make you a negative person. When others try to change your behavior, you will retreat further into denying the need for change. Accepting the negativity of your habits is the first step. If you are unwilling to examine your own behavior, you will never accept it as negative. Accepting how your behavior affects other people will allow you to identify negative behaviors you are unaware of. Examining the source of each behavior is not as important as identifying the triggers of the behaviors.

We can trigger positive habits as easily as negative ones. We form positive habits from our knowledge. Negative habits come from our beliefs. We continue negative habits because we do not see them as negative. If you smoke, overeat, or have another habit you know is unhealthy, you will avoid examining it. You convince yourself the behavior makes you happy, regardless of the health consequences. These unexamined habits will eventually become addictions you cannot easily change.

Addictions are dangerous for us and the people in our lives. They negatively affect our health, shorten our lives, and decrease the quality of our lives. As behaviors go, they are the most destructive. Addictions can range from alcohol to gambling, but any repeated negative behavior can become an addiction. An unexamined reality is the leading cause of our addictions. Only others can see the damage we are doing to ourselves. Even if we recognize the damage we are doing, it may be too late to recover from it.

One addiction many people have is hurrying through life. If you are often in a hurry, always trying to find shortcuts, and get frustrated when others are not going fast enough, you are hurrying through life. The destination you are speeding to will never arrive because you are always speeding to the next destination. You are speeding your way to your death. Ignoring your addiction to speed will lead to ignoring the reality of your health. You will miss the genuine cause of your health problems while you are running through life.

Our ability to ignore reality can allow us to avoid temptations. Ignoring reality can be dangerous, but we can use it to control our addictions. Removing temptations from our environment is one of the best ways to ignore them. We can focus our attention on more positive behaviors and ignore the triggers to our negative habits. Accepting the reality of our behavior is the best way to change it. We can use our ability to ignore reality to avoid and eliminate our unhealthy behaviors.

We can only examine the behaviors of others and not what triggered them to act. Court cases look at the reasons for people's behaviors, but they are not usually relevant or accurate to why people act as they do. Viewing the behavior of others through your own unexamined behaviors will lead to incorrect conclusions. In a courtroom, an incorrect conclusion can ruin people's lives.

We can only judge people by their behavior because that is the only option most of the time. Pretending we can see the motivations of others in their behavior only rarely leads to the truth. If we focused less on punishing people for their behavior and more on helping them accept their behavior as a problem, we could help more people with their behavioral problems.

Noticing appropriate behavior is just as important as noticing inappropriate behavior. Children misbehave because they are still learning the consequences of their actions. As adults, we no longer have this excuse. Inappropriate behavior should embarrass us as adults. Because of the power structures of many societies, we accept inappropriate behavior from people in power. Some people think of their inappropriate behavior as an entertaining part of their personality. Others are completely unaware of their own behavior. Only when their behavior affects something they care about will they examine it.

When I see others behaving negatively, I know they are miserable. If you care about yourself, you will care about the world around you. If you are miserable inside, you will treat the outside world horribly. The more miserable you are, the worse your behavior will become. When trying to help others rid themselves of negative behaviors, we should not constantly reprimand the same behavior. They will only change their behavior when they experience the negative consequences of it. Working with them to see these consequences is the only way they will positively change.

Justifying Our Bad Behavior

*"I behave like everyone else does, but
it's bad behavior when I do it. If I treated
people nicely, they wouldn't know it was
me. I'm just a bad person. I can't change
who I am."*

Reality Denial

*"I treat people the same way I expect
them to treat me. Some people are
unaware of their effect on other people. I
try to avoid those people when I can. When
people behave badly, I know there is
something making them not care about
others. Inappropriate behavior is how they
show this."*

Reality Acceptance

Justifying our bad behavior seems to be a favorite pastime for many people. We tell ourselves being late to work justifies our speeding. We justify staying up too late to finish watching our favorite show. Whatever goal we consider most important takes priority over our behavior. If you accomplish your goal, you justify your behavior. In reality, your behavior is completely unjustified and unhealthy for you and the other people in your life.

Our justifications happen all the time. People justify jaywalking, ignoring others in need, and many other negative behaviors. We justify these small behaviors by their insignificance. We ignore them from others, so we assume others are ignoring us. Most people only focus on their own lives and do not notice other people. Even when negative behavior is unnoticed by others, it is still unhealthy behavior.

Our prison systems are full of people who could not justify their unhealthy behavior. Most times, they could not afford a good enough attorney to justify their actions. Prisons do not concern themselves with preventing bad behavior. The law deals with punishing people for their illegal actions, not rehabilitating them. When we send people to prison, they can learn more unhealthy behaviors. Over population, racism, and underfunding rehabilitation efforts contribute significantly to the problem. We send people to prison to remove and hide them from society, not to rehabilitate them back into society.

Because our behavior is legal, or no one catches us does not justify it. We rationalize our behavior as if it does not directly harm others. Especially if no one is there to witness our behavior, we declare ourselves free of guilt. Unwitnessed bad behavior is still bad behavior. Cheating is an unjustifiable choice, even if they do not catch you. You are cheating someone else out of an accomplishment you did not earn. Considering your behavior innocent because it is not a crime denies its effect on you and others.

People who call themselves or others call them lazy are actually unhappy. We call others lazy when we are unhappy with our lives and looking for others to blame. No one is lazy. What appears as laziness is a lack of enthusiasm for life. We do not want to spend our days doing little to improve our lives, but our emotions will not let us change for the better. Working on your life represents confronting all your failures, which led to your current misery. Claiming you or someone else is lazy is easier than dealing with the failures and traumas of your past. Your negative attitude about yourself or others is a sign of your misery. Justifying your negative behavior will only make things worse.

Many people see anonymity as a justification for bad behavior. Being anonymous allows us to ignore the consequences of our actions. Most people ignore anonymous behavior from others. This does not justify it, but it allows anonymous people to vent their frustrations on others without consequences. It is a role-playing game they play to entertain themselves regardless of the harm they cause to others. They justify their behavior by its entertainment value to them.

Good and bad behaviors are not all or nothing. Kind of good behavior is still good behavior. Equating all behavior as justified or unjustified leads to over reactions from others. People see others as heroes or villains without seeing the middle. Without understanding other's motives, you cannot judge them. Continuous planned bad behavior is worse than a singular unplanned bad behavior. The better or worse behavior you witness in others, the better you can judge their behavior overall.

Other People Exist

"People have told me I can be
obnoxious and loud. I don't even notice
people around me most of the time. Why
can't they just ignore me like I do them?"

Reality Denial

"I am always aware when other
people are near me. If I'm in their way, I
want to be aware of it before they are.
When I'm in a room and some people are
ignoring other people, I want to
acknowledge them."

Reality Acceptance

"Other People Exist" may seem like a simple-minded phrase. I might as well say only humans will read this book. Reminding you that other people exist is about reminding your brain. People surround us most of our lives, but how often do we acknowledge their existence? These people we ignore still exist and affect our lives. Most of us do not see them unless they interact with us directly. We notice people who create positive or negative emotions in us more than those who are more neutral. Ignoring these other people ignores their existence and our behavior toward them.

How you interact with other people is entirely up to you. Pretending they do not exist does not make them go away. Recognizing that other people exist is a statistically logical statement. All humans will have to deal with at least a portion of other humans throughout their lives. The more we accept this, the more connected we can be with one another. As soon as we say we will only recognize those humans who agree with us, who live close to us, or who drink the same soft drinks we do, we cease to live cohesive and connected lives. Other people do not exist because we want them to exist or believe they exist, they just exist.

Coming together as a world community will not be easy, but it is necessary to avoid as many conflicts as possible. We must make compromises among all communities. We can live without acknowledging other people's existence, but we will have conflicts with other people throughout our lives. This will have negative repercussions for ourselves and the other people. Allowing both good and bad connections with one another will allow us all to accept others into our lives and thoughts.

If two people want to sit in a one-person chair, only one can sit with his butt touching the seat at once. The two people can fight to sit in the chair first, or they can share the chair at different times. Compromise is the key to both living together in a one-chair world. Not compromising will lead to constant conflict. We avoid people we have conflicts with, and the conflicts become worse. Connecting with more people in your life will lead to fewer conflicts.

Acknowledging the existence of every other person on earth is not a realistic goal. Recognizing the existence of others is acknowledging people you come into contact with. If you can talk to them, see them, hear them, or interact with them, you merely need to accept them into your consciousness. If other people think you are worthy of acknowledgment as a person, so are other people. Acknowledgments must go both ways.

Everyone who is not you is an "other." This includes your family and friends, but most people do not see them this way. Many people use this as an excuse to separate themselves from specific people. If we disagree with others, deny they exist, or fear them, we will place them in our minds as other people. We can even see them as inhuman. If we have to spend time with them, we will treat them with hostility or ignore them.

The hostility we show others can lead to an argument or fight with them. It is more about seeing those people as "others" than the disagreement itself. If we are the ones being hostile to others, we are denying their existence in our minds. They are other people who we do not care about, dismiss, and treat as enemies. We scrutinize everything they say, do, and are. They may feel the same about us, but we do not care about them enough to find out. In our minds, they feel the same about us because they are heartless jerks. The hate we feel is not harming them, but it is definitely harming us.

When we judge others, we are judging ourselves. If you do not care about others, you do not care about yourself. Instead of blaming our misery on ourselves, we blame others. We judge other people by our surface level views of them. They represent ideas and views we hate. Hate of any kind is a negative emotion that will keep you from being happy and healthy. If your enemies knew they were having this effect on you, they would either not care or delight at making you miserable.

When we look at other people, we view them through our experiences, beliefs, and knowledge of our world. What we are missing is a knowledge of their world. We can see movies about despicable people and sympathize with them. We do this because we see life from their point of view. Real people are not heroes or villains. The people we see as "other" are not actual people in our minds. They are other people who we never get to know. When we judge them without knowing them, we keep them as villains. We do not want to get to know them as genuine people.

Sometimes, we get to know other people and we still dislike them. Their view on life, behavior, and attitude makes us feel negative when we are around them. If we constantly feel this way around them, we must remove ourselves from them as much as we can. They are viewing those who do not act as they do as "others." They focus narrowly on their beliefs and reject others who do not believe as they do. In their mind, we are other people who they do not care about. We should not make the same mistake they are making by viewing them as stereotypes. Talk to them as people, not the stereotypes they present to others.

Accept other people as you would want them to accept you. Thinking, acting, and looking different from you is not enough to reject them as people. The assumptions you are making about them would be just as incorrect as the assumptions they could make about you. Our normal response should be to accept other people. Only by getting to know them can we judge them. When we get to know them, they stop being "others" and start being other people who exist in our lives.

Reality Accepting Exercise:

Notice the unhealthy behavior around you. Are there people creating an unnecessarily stressful situation, being unsafe to others, or being angry at everyone? As you see these things, think about a time in the past when you acted in the same or similar way. Was there ever a logical reason you acted as you did? (Hint – the answer is always "no") What can you learn from this unhealthy behavior to stop you from behaving this way in the future? What happened before you behaved as you did that led to your behavior?

How you behave toward others is how they will perceive you. We have justifications in our heads for our behavior, but they only see our behavior. Behaving well involves being able to view yourself from other people's perspectives. You should know your behavior and its effect on other people.

Chapter 20
Social Skills

*"I don't enjoy going to places that get
all uptight about cussing and letting me be
who I am. I like to hang out in bars and
parties that get out of control. That's
where I'm truly accepted for who I am."*

Reality Denial

*"I usually know what behavior is
acceptable in different social interactions.
I would never act in a way that made other
people uncomfortable. If I do something
that is out of the ordinary for me, it's with
people who know me well."*

Reality Acceptance

Developing social skills is just as important as developing any other skill. If you are not comfortable interacting with others, you will not do so. Diverse social interactions will allow you to develop more diverse social skills. Learning what is acceptable is as important as learning what is unacceptable. If you have better social skills than other people, it is up to you to guide them in the interaction. Having underdeveloped social skills will lead to negative behaviors and failed relationships.

The first place we learn social skills is playing with other kids when we are young. The playground becomes just as important as the classroom. Kids who interact well with others will become popular, while kids who do not begin a lifetime of negative behaviors. Bullies, shy kids, misfits, and kids with low self-esteem will result. Instead of playing with other kids, they isolate themselves and can develop anti-social behaviors.

Much of developing social skills is about observation. I was a shy kid, but I observed others. I saw their positive and negative interactions and learned from them. It would be years before I came out of my shell, but I learned positive social skills. One of my greatest skills was listening. Most of my life, people told me things they told no one else because I would listen without interrupting. I observed the social cues many people missed.

Some people do not know why they behave as they do. Our social skills depend on observing others and acting accordingly. When you treat every interaction the same way, you are ignoring the behavior of others. Thinking about what you do is just as important as doing it. We must balance actions and reactions with other people. A balanced conversation will lead to a positive exchange between people. If you are unaware of why you are having the conversation, you are not a balanced member.

Your social skills will affect your behavior positively or negatively. If you value social skills, your behavior will benefit. If you deny the importance of social skills, your behavior will reflect it. Your social interactions will be a mixture of positive and negative behaviors you cannot distinguish between. You will misinterpret most social interactions, which will lead to your misbehaving. Your misbehavior will only stand out to others, but not to you. We feel comfortable telling kids about their misbehavior, but we feel uncomfortable telling adults.

Misbehavior will only get worse as we age. If other people do not point out your misbehavior, you will never learn from it. Your behavior will continue to get worse. Some people focus their energy on environments more accepting of misbehavior. They see their success as more important than positive interactions with others. They have success, but few positive relationships with others.

People who develop negative social skills are not bad people. They are usually unaware of their effect on others. Other people do not want to interact with them because most interactions are unpleasant or awkward. Their social skills can be underdeveloped for many reasons. I have found it easier than most to talk to these awkward people. This was me for much of my life, so I can relate to them. I do not judge them by their behavior. My interest in them is as people. Everyone has an interesting story, even if they tell it awkwardly.

Relating to people with diminished social skills is important to helping them improve their skills. Over time, they will learn from positive interactions. If they have no positive interactions, they will not improve. The more they can practice positive social interactions, the more they will improve. Playing an instrument well takes many hours of playing badly.

Many environments are not conducive to positive social interactions. These are environments such as restaurants, parties, bars, live events, and at work. We think of these places as perfect for social interactions, but they are not. The focus of these environments is on something other than interacting with others. If you have friends you only interact with at these places, you are more acquaintances than friends.

We all want to interact well with others, but our social skills may prevent us from affectively doing so. Allowing everyone to take part in social interactions is an important part of having diverse interactions. If you are skilled at social interactions, help others who are not. The most interesting voices are the ones we rarely hear.

Empathy

*"Why should I care about other
people when they don't care about me? If
somebody needs help, I assume other
people will do something. I can never tell
if people are just whining about nothing,
or they actually need something."*

Reality Denial

*"I care about other people and can
usually tell if they need help. People's
emotions come out in their actions. I can
tell how people feel before they have
admitted it to themselves."*

Reality Acceptance

Empathy is an important social skill. People who do not care about others do not care about themselves. You can care about those people, but they will not see themselves as worthy of empathy. They may eventually open up to caring about others and themselves, so it is important to show them empathy. When you are empathetic to others, you have earned the right to hear their story. They may not want to tell their story, but you have shown you will be receptive to it without judgment.

People do not have to be completely selfish or completely altruistic. Just as a moderate politician is more balanced, a person who is only selfish or only altruistic is not living a balanced life. Thinking only of others is just as unhealthy as only thinking of yourself. You cannot do good for others if you neglect your own health. If you are happy and healthy in your life, you can help others who are not. Empathizing with others is different from feeling their emotions. You are feeling empathy for their emotional problems, but it is dangerous to feel their unhealthy emotions. Helping others should add to your happiness and health.

Some people are proud of their selfishness. They proudly display clothing, bumper stickers, and other self-aggrandizing signs of their love for themselves. These displays are examples of their inner insecurities. If a company advertises their product, they are insecure about whether their product will sell. Self-centered people do not think about others long enough to empathize with them. We can try to accept reality on their behalf, but it will not work. They must recognize their insecurities for themselves.

I care about strangers. I have empathy for strangers, even though I do not know them. Even someone who is displaying destructive behavior receives my full empathy. Destructive behavior does not make someone a bad person. You can feel empathy for people you strongly dislike. Their destructive behavior is nothing compared to the inner turmoil they are putting themselves through. We can never know the reasons for a stranger's behaviors. Empathizing with them is the best way to get to know them.

We can all be happier and healthier if we add more empathy into our lives. Empathizing with others is a behavior that will only add value to our lives. The more we empathize with others, the more they will empathize with us. It is a habit that will serve you well in your life. Just as you must practice physical skills, you must practice empathy to exercise your social skills. The positive effects on your mental health will lead to positive effects on your physical health.

SEE MORE EXAMPLES AT:

realityacceptance.com/category/behavior/empathy/

Reality Accepting Exercise:

Notice the social interactions around you throughout your day. Are there certain locations, people, or times of day that have more positive interactions? How many people do you have positive social interactions with? Do you find more positive or negative interactions? What is the difference between people who are more or less social? Do more social people appear happier than those who are less social?

Having positive social interactions relates closely to how empathetic you are toward others. If you care about others less, you will be less social with them. People who do not engage with others often expect most social interactions to be negative. People who interact positively with others regularly know that most people will interact positively if you are positive to them first. If you show you care about others, they will usually care about you.

Chapter 21
Unhealthy Behavior

Lying to Yourself and Others

*"I wouldn't have any
accomplishments if I didn't lie about them.
No one would ever date me, my family
would disown me, and I definitely wouldn't
be the top salesman at my company."*

Reality Denial

*"I have never been a good liar. The
truth is always much more interesting than
lies. Telling yourself you have to lie to
others tells them you don't trust them with
the truth. Most BS artists are only fooling
themselves."*

Reality Acceptance

Lying is not a natural behavior. Other species deceive others
to survive, but only humans lie to others for far less than
survival. We have to teach infants to lie. They see their parents
and others lying to each other and they emulate the behavior.
If they get out of trouble by lying, the lying behavior becomes
re-enforced. Children absorb the behaviors of those around
them. They emulate what they see. Gestures and patterns of
speech develop in the children come directly from their
parents. You tell your child not to lie while lying to others.

The child is much more influenced by your behavior than your words.

Lying is a destructive habit that only gets worse with time. The more you lie to others and get away with it, the better your skill at lying gets. When you lie to other people, you are not respecting them as people. You believe they cannot handle the truth, or you just do not want to tell them the truth. Many people justify lying to others with faulty reasoning or denying the impact they have on other people. Lying is a skill that degrades your life the more you practice it.

People good at lying are good at ignoring the consequences of their lies. They see the lie as a line of dialog they are delivering as an actor. They are proud of themselves the more lies they get away with telling. The game of lying distorts their view of other people. People become game pieces they manipulate to get what they want. Their self-esteem is high, but their care for others is low. Living fast and dying young is their motto because they ignore consequences. They are running away from their lies and toward a premature death from the negative effects on their health.

It is easier to lie to strangers than to people you know. Lies depend on other people's beliefs. If others believe you are lying, you will have a hard time lying to them. If others believe you are telling the truth, you will have an easier time lying to them. When judging whether others are lying, it is best to judge the information they are presenting rather than trusting them. Judging other people's behavior will not tell you whether they are lying. A talented liar will behave the same as a person who is telling the truth. Others who do not behave as you expect might appear to lie when they are not.

Despite what some people believe, you cannot judge whether a person is lying based on their behavior.

Some adults and children do not have entrenched beliefs about what others say. They question everything. If you tell them a lie that others accept, they question it. It is not socially acceptable in many circumstances to question others. It is especially unacceptable to point out if someone is lying. When you do not have these beliefs about what is socially acceptable, you do not hold yourself back from pointing out obvious lies. People and children who do not have these beliefs are the closest thing we have to a reliable lie detector. They are the enemy of the talented liar, but are exactly what they need.

Insincere Smiles

Some people do not smile unless you tell them to do so. Others have a smile on their face all day. Most of us are somewhere in the middle. We think the person who does not smile is angry or sad. Smiling at everyone shows you care about them. It is polite and acceptable behavior, but is insincere much of the time. Smiling for strangers is putting on a dishonest smile. A smile comes from within you. It shows how you are feeling. It is not something you put on for other people. If you are looking for honesty, you would be better off trusting the person who is not smiling.

Insincere people put on smiling faces and are friendly to people they want to attract or impress. On the job, we tell employees to be pleasant, so customers will buy more. Neighbors wave at each other to avoid negative behavior from one another. All the people in commercials are insincere. No one can be excited about dish soap. Insincere people act pleasantly so they can get what they want from others. It is a socially accepted lie.

Actors are people who we pay to be insincere. If acting were real, it would not be acting. Many people considered the best actors are the most insincere people. When they are not acting, they do not know who they are as people. They can only act on stage or on the screen and, eventually, in life. They become the persona of whatever character they are currently playing. The actual person inside disappears while they are acting.

You should be the same person in private as you are in public. The further these two things are from one another, the further you are from accepting reality. If you can only feel appreciated by putting on a show, you are an insecure person. I am a happy person most of the time, but I only smile when I sincerely feel like doing so. Being insincere to other people is lying to them about your genuine feelings.

SEE MORE EXAMPLES AT:

realityacceptance.com/category/behavior/unhealthy-behavior/

realityacceptance.com/category/behavior/lying/

realityacceptance.com/category/behavior/insincerity/

Hidden Motives

*"I went to my mom's house the other
day to ask her for money. I took some
flowers with me from my neighbor's house
to soften her up. She looked at me with the
flowers and said, 'What do you want
now?' I said, 'Can't a son do something
nice for his mom?' She said, in my case,
'No.'"*

Reality Denial

*"I can always tell when someone does
me a favor expecting something in return.
It's usually the same people who have
done it before. If I do someone a favor, it's
because I care about them. I don't expect
anything in return."*

Reality Acceptance

Hiding your motives is lying to others. People hide their motives so they can trick others into giving them what they want. They hide their motive because the motives are not sincere. A child agrees to make her bed to cover up something she is hiding in the bed. Some people can be unaware of their own hidden motives, but most people know what they are doing. Either way, they are not being sincere with those they are manipulating.

I was in high school ~~when I got a part-time job~~ when I got a part-time job as a phone solicitor. We would sit at tables with phones and call from a random list of names and phone numbers. There was a page long script we would read verbatim to the people on the phone. We would insinuate they had won a prize, but the real prize was a visit to their house by a salesperson who would attempt to sell them even more. It was an obvious example of hidden motives. After that job was over, I vowed never to do anything like sales ever again.

An example of hidden motives is when a company donates money or merchandise to a charity or other worthy cause. The company will often create ads to announce the good deed so they can get sufficient publicity from it. Only a few people notice the obvious motives of the company because most of us do not pay close attention. Ads use hidden motives when they entertain, inform, or emotionally manipulate the audience into forgetting they are watching an ad.

People think they are hiding their motives well, but they are completely obvious most of the time. A salesperson treats you nicely and offers you free samples, but ignores you as soon as he knows you are not buying anything from him. People barely hide their true motives to get what they want. If the salesperson cannot easily fool you, he moves on to the next sale. Hidden motives hurt both the deceiver and those they are deceiving.

SEE MORE EXAMPLES AT:

realityacceptance.com/category/behavior/hidden-motives/

Revenge

*"Someday, I'm going to take revenge
on all my enemies. I have many enemies
and I will never forget what they did to me.
They may think I have forgiven them by
now, but they are wrong."*

Reality Denial

*"When people mistreat me, I know
their lives are miserable. The horrible
thing they did to me is nothing compared
to the misery of their lives. I'm not going
to make myself miserable by hating them."*

Reality Acceptance

Revenge is a dish best unserved. I changed this cliche phrase to point out the reality of revenge. Revenge on other people is about you. You feel like a victim yourself, so you want to make others a victim. Most of the time, you are far less of a victim than you think. Even when you are the recipient of negative behavior, your thoughts of revenge exceed the level of victimization you received. Seeking revenge on others is an unhealthy behavior that never turns out like you plan.

My dad was someone who got along with most other people and did whatever he could to help them. If you had wronged him, he had a vengeful side that would come out. He would make sure you knew you had wronged him. He always remembered what other people did to him and treated them differently. His revenge was not in the form of retaliating against others, but not respecting or helping them. They were off his list of people who deserved his respect or help. I must admit, I take after my dad in this way. It is the closest thing to revenge that comes out in my behavior.

Seeking revenge is a behavior that gets worse the more you practice it. It is assessing a situation, judging others, and enacting a punishment all in one. Instead of logically assessing the situation, reserving judgment until you have all the facts, and resolving the situation through a true understanding of it, you go right to revenge. Revenge becomes a way of life. Like any other unhealthy behavior, revenge never leads to a happy conclusion.

People seek revenge on others because they see themselves as a victim. Someone or a group of people mistreated them. Their desire for revenge comes from seeing themselves as a lifelong victim. The revenge tells others they will no longer be a victim. Their motives come from their beliefs about other people. Insecurities prevent them from looking beyond their beliefs to assess the reality of the situation. We don't carry out our most vengeful thoughts because of these insecurities. Even without enacting the revenge, we have carried out the damage to our own health.

Forgiving others is about forgiving ourselves for being a victim. Even if someone wronged us, it is still in our best interest to forgive them. If they behave badly, they will pay the price of living a miserable and unhealthy life. We should not join them by damaging our own health. Revenge is an unhealthy practice for everyone involved in it.

The Blame Game

> *"If I'm messed up at all, it's because
> of my parents. They never taught me what
> a good relationship looks like, so I've
> never had one. There's nothing I can do
> about it now because they're both dead."*

Reality Denial

> *"I never blame other people for
> things I do wrong. When I think about it, it
> is always my own actions that caused
> things to go wrong. I don't blame a person
> who is blind for tripping me with his cane
> if I was running past him. Blaming others
> is just redirecting your anger toward
> yourself."*

Reality Acceptance

We blame others to deflect from our own guilt. If something goes wrong, our first thought is to assess our guilt in the incident. If we find others to blame, we lash out at them to prove our innocence. It is an unnecessary overreaction most times. If we are partially guilty, we may exaggerate our innocence more. Blaming others is about deflecting blame from ourselves.

Most incidents have multiple causes. There is no single factor or blame to assign. We can accept the reality of the incident without assigning blame. Blaming others is an attempt to simplify an incident. We assign blame because we assume there is a guilty party who caused the incident. There are few incidents we can view with this amount of simplicity.

A group can assign blame to a single person if it will deflect from multiple guilty parties. Why should everyone involved receive punishment when one person can take the blame for the rest? The person who gets singled out is usually lower in status and expendable in the eyes of the group. Anyone who allows the injustice to occur denies the reality of the situation. They are not acting ethically or logically.

There are many reasons we assign blame to others. The primary reason is we do not want others to blame us. Most of the time, blaming others is unnecessary and unfounded. If a few people are to blame for errors in judgment, we should not punish them. Instead, we should educate them, so they do not make the error again. The sooner all involved accept the reality of the situation, the quicker people can move on to more important issues and prevent errors in the future.

Gossips

"I know everything that is going on in our office. From such gossip as who is cheating on their spouse, who is lying to their boss, and how many times we have all almost lost our jobs, I know everything. I know things before they happen around here."

Reality Denial

"I don't listen to gossip in our office. Most of the time, it turns out to be a false rumor. If something bad is going to happen to me I don't know about, I'm not going to worry myself before it happens."

Reality Acceptance

We gossip about others for many reasons. Whether it is jealousy, revenge, boredom, or wanting to be the center of attention, we gossip to declare ourselves superior to others. We base gossip on rumors and unproven accusations about others. People create gossip from coincidence, beliefs, speculation, and lies. It can ruin the lives of others and tarnish the reputation of the gossiper. It is unhealthy behavior that leads to negative consequences for everyone involved.

People only gossip about acquaintances. If they cared about the people they were gossiping about, they would not gossip about them. Seeing these people from a distance allows the gossiper to speculate wildly and add to the drama of the gossip. We gossip to entertain and leave our audiences wanting more. Gathering more gossip becomes key to growing our popularity as a gossip. The people who listen to and believe the gossip allow the gossiper to continue. They are accomplices in the crime.

People gossip about others until they are the recipient of someone else's gossip. The game is only fun if you are in charge of all the moves. As soon as we become the subject of the gossip, we see the negative side of our behavior. We will hopefully stop gossiping about others when we see how it affected us. Viewing others as characters to gossip about is not viewing them as people. Whenever we view others as inhuman, we lose our humanity.

SEE MORE EXAMPLES AT:

realityacceptance.com/category/behavior/gossips/

Reality Accepting Exercise:

Think back on your life. How many examples of unhealthy behavior can you think of from your past? Did anyone call you out on your behavior? Do you remember more times when others called you out or when no one else knew how you behaved? Was your behavior worse with strangers or people you knew? Did you have a justification in your mind for your behavior? Has your behavior improved as you have gotten older?

People behave based on their inner emotional state. If you have undealt with emotional problems, they will show up as unhealthy behavioral problems. Changing your behavior involves changing how you view other people. We behave badly to others when we feel they are behaving badly toward us. Use the unhealthy behavior of others to judge their inner emotional state. You can do the same with your own emotional state. The more you understand your own behavior, the more you can understand others.

Chapter 22
Exclusionary Behavior

"I belong to an exclusive country club. We only allow members we deem worthy of living up to our high standards. If one of our members breaks our rules, we make sure he and no one else in his family may come back."

Reality Denial

"They have excluded me from enough groups to know what that's like. I never want to be a part of a group doing that to other people. Most of the times they excluded me, I have been glad they didn't trap me into hanging out with such narrow-minded people."

Reality Acceptance

Some behaviors purposely exclude us from others. We avoid behaving in ways we believe are unacceptable and behave negatively toward others to discourage them from behaving in these ways. The more we exclude them from our lives, the less social we become. We isolate ourselves from most people and live an acceptable but miserable life. Most of our behavior is deliberate and purposeful. Some people may be unaware of their own behavior, but they have taken cues from others who are. Excluding others from your life is excluding yourself from most people.

In elementary school, a group I was in excluded a friend of mine from the group. I do not remember why they excluded him, but I remember he was asking me for help, and I ignored him. This was one of the few times in my young life I was part of a group of kids. I did not want to jeopardize my place in the group by helping him. They eventually kicked me out of the group when they got to know me. It was an excellent lesson about why excluding others is harmful for everyone. It was the first of many times I would learn this life lesson.

Feeling good about ourselves should not include excluding others. If our self-worth comes from seeing ourselves in an exclusive and privileged group, we are excluding others. We justify our behavior because we are keeping what we see as the natural order of things. We deserve the privileges and exclude others who do not. In reality, we exclude others to maintain our privileges. We cannot imagine our lives without these privileges. If you never give up your privileges, you will never fall in love, make friends, or experience any part of life requiring you to be vulnerable. Enjoy the solitude.

Excluding others is unhealthy for the excluder and the excluded. We separate people into us and them. This can lead to behaviors as small as snubbing someone else or as large as declaring war on another group. These collective behaviors will develop into exclusive groups, secret information, and exclusionary rules. When groups exclude themselves from others, they eliminate positive interactions with outside groups. Membership in these groups will lead to unhealthy behaviors and thinking.

We can find examples of exclusionary behavior throughout history. Discrimination against minority groups and people who were different happened well before we kept historical records. The reason this still happens today is minority groups rarely gain power or control over dominant cultures. The main thing current dominant groups have accomplished is keeping their dominant status. As we become more diverse as a global community, these exclusionary behaviors will become less acceptable. We will never remove them from all societies, but they will be far less widespread.

SEE MORE EXAMPLES AT:

realityacceptance.com/category/behavior/exclusionary-behavior/

Pride & Shame

*"I am proud of my ancestors for
building this country where I can live free.
It's a shame people always have to focus
on slavery, racism, sexism, and
homophobia. They were of their time. Get
over it!"*

Reality Denial

*"I don't consider pride a good thing.
I definitely don't consider shame a good
thing. It is not for you to decide whether
you or a group you are in deserve praise.
You should earn praise through your
actions, not just by being yourself or a part
of a group."*

Reality Acceptance

Humans use pride and shame to regulate the behavior of others. We can also use them to exclude others. Shame is an obvious way to exclude others, but we use pride for the same purpose. We often view pride and shame as complete opposites. We are full of pride or shame with no middle ground. This is a form of extreme thinking. Pride is different from dignity. Pride separates us from others. We are proud of what we accomplished only because others did not do so.

Respecting ourselves is as important as respecting others. If we think we deserve more respect than others, we usually have an inflated view of ourselves. Having a good respect for your accomplishments is healthy for your self-esteem. Respecting yourself over others is unhealthy and will lead to pride. You do not need pride in yourself to have a healthy self-image. Our greatest accomplishments come when we help others and encourage them to do the same. Pride is an unnecessary part of accomplishing something.

We all must be able to work with other people. A group thinking themselves deserving of more pride than others will separate themselves from other groups. All groups deserve equal respect. Otherwise, groups will only have pride in their own accomplishments. "We're number one!" is a disturbing chant which allows groups to see themselves as better than other groups. This is unhealthy for everyone.

Shaming others is especially unhealthy for society. We shame others to force them into feeling guilty about their behavior. Guilt and shame are not the same. We feel guilty about behavior we regret. We shame others who do not adhere to our societal rules. Feeling the shame requires social pressure from the outside. If you have compassion for yourself, the shame will not work. It will still exclude you, but you will know you have nothing to feel ashamed about.

I am a vegan most of the time. Some people would say you are not a vegan unless you are always a vegan. This form of shaming does not work on me. I am not proud of being a vegan. I am glad I am a vegan because I feel better when I eat a vegan diet. Accepting shame or pride to please others is rarely necessary and will lead to unhealthy behaviors. For our own health, we should avoid them both.

SEE MORE EXAMPLES AT:

realityacceptance.com/category/behavior/pride-shame/

Gender Roles

*"As the man of the house, I make all
the money, decide what is best for my
family, and give all the orders. My wife
takes care of the kids and cleans the house.
This is how is has worked for generations
in my family. Why change what ain't
broke?"*

Reality Denial

*"I don't accept most of the gender
roles my parents thrust upon me. My dad
and mom both seem miserable in the
patriarchal roles that their parents gave
them. Why would I follow outdated rules
from unhappy people?"*

Reality Acceptance

Societies usually establish gender roles when we are kids. I was a boy, so they expected me to behave like other boys. Much of the time, I did not want to behave like them. They were immature, illogical, and negative. Whenever I attempted to behave like them, I felt only negative emotions. I can now see I was correct in my avoidance of these behaviors. They were not healthy for me or any of the other kids.

They established our gender roles in whatever society we live in. Most societies have accepted the dominance of men over women. We developed these dominant behaviors as we evolved from apes. We are no longer dominating with our strength, but with power. Males still outnumber females in positions of power. This is changing, but only in areas that accept the inequities of the past. These accepted gender roles were not logical thousands or years ago, and they are especially not logical today.

Women accept more realities than men because life forces them to accept them. Girls must accept the realities of their periods, pregnancy, body image, and many other realities of living in a patriarchal society. Most politicians and leaders are men, so they do not accept the reality of basic human rights for women. Most men find this inequity acceptable because of the privileges they experience throughout their lives. These privileges shield them from the realities women deal with every day. This greater acceptance of reality has led to women living longer and healthier lives.

Societies with more women in positions of power are more advanced societies. The patriarchal societies of the past will seem as outdated as slavery, monarchies, and genocide. The less we allow our beliefs about our gender roles to control our behaviors, the more we will accept the positive roles we all play in society. Toxic masculinity and gender inequality have taken their toll on societies, but it does not doom us to continue these practices. Your positive role in society has much less to do with your assigned gender than your acceptance of reality.

LGBTQ Issues

*"I don't have the energy to worry
about what they want me to call them this
week. Their pronoun is of no concern to
me. What's next? Are they going to force
me to refer to my dog as a duck? Why is
this just now becoming as issue?"*

Reality Denial

*"LGBTQ issues affect all of us. If you
think these issues affect no one in your life,
you are ignoring most of the people in
your life. Those of us who don't adhere to
the patriarchal standards of sexual
orientation and gender identity are most
people."*

Reality Acceptance

Reality for people in the LGBTQ (lesbian, gay, bisexual, transgender, and queer) community does not differ from reality for other people. They deserve the same respect we all do. Some people mistakenly view LGBTQ issues as behavioral because they only see the behavior that they find objectionable. People's mental images of themselves do not match the bodies they inhabit. We exclude them from society for not accepting our expectations for their lives. They accept the reality of themselves, but society does not.

People in the LGBTQ community are less violent, hateful, or discriminatory than most other people are. Why are they treated as outsiders in most societies? People fear what they do not understand. If you grew up feeling comfortable in your body, attracted to acceptable partners, and living up to the expectations of mainstream society, you may not understand those who do not. If you think this describes you, you are lying to yourself. You are living an acceptable life dictated by society. You may never question these expectations until the end of your life when you regret not being true to yourself.

We spend much of our lives lying to ourselves. We tell ourselves we are living our happiest and healthiest lives when we are not. Many people in the LGBTQ community lie to themselves until they accept the reality of their own lies. When any of us stops lying to ourselves, a flood of positive and negative emotions can overwhelm us. We are regretful of the years we lied to ourselves, but we are excited and apprehensive for the future. How will our family and friends react when they find out their perception of us was a lie? Many people in the LGBTQ community know how their family and friends will react. It is the reason they lied to themselves and others for so long.

We discriminate against the LGBTQ community because we believe ourselves justified. Unprovoked negative behavior toward others is never logical or ethical. We take our frustrations out on other people, but we are mad at them for accepting a reality we deny. Realizing the true source of our negative emotions and behavior is key to removing our exclusionary behaviors from society. We need to accept the reality of our own behavior and help others accept it for themselves.

Race and Racism

*"I'm not racist, but I don't see why
we should treat someone special just
because of how my ancestors treated their
ancestors. I've never seen a racist
interaction in my life. What is the
problem?"*

Reality Denial

*"Race is not real, but racism is. The
only way to stop racism is to combat it
when we see it. This includes in person
and when we see that certain racial groups
are more discriminated against than
others. You can only ignore or deny
statistics. Numbers change from area to
area, but they are always disproportionate
to the dominant culture in control of that
area."*

Reality Acceptance

Race does not exist, but racism does. The origins of racism go back to the first humans who saw themselves as different from other humans because of physical traits. The terms race and racism are fairly recent social constructs in human history. Scientists "legitimized" the concept by creating unscientific studies, showing how we could separate people into races. The physical differences among people do not affect their ability to learn, grow, teach, or live their life unless they must deal with racist ideologies. Racism is a creation of bias, illogical thinking, and prejudice.

The concept of race persists in societies who do not believe in fundamental aspects of reality. Religions, economic institutions, competitive organizations, and other groups allowed this myth to fester. If a group of people accept one myth, they will accept other myths. This does not mean racism is a myth. Racist ideologies are decreasing as time goes on; however, this only means people must hide racist ideologies. Those affected by them are fully aware of the reality of racism. They experience the illogical behavior that has no other explanation beyond racism.

We view racism as an ethical issue, but it is more of a logical issue. There is no scientific or logical explanation for accepting the concept of race. Any argument that does not accept all humans as deserving of human rights is illogical. Societies who still accept racist policies are intellectually inferior to more advanced societies. We cannot rid societies of racism without eliminating the illogical ideologies that allowed the racism. People who denounce racism as unethical may not accept the illogical origins of the racism. If we do not accept all of reality, we cannot fix problems in society such as racism.

Most racist policies in societies continue because of the racist ideologies of those in power. Racist policies will not end without removing the policies of racist politicians. These can be current politicians or politicians from the past. As long as their policies stand, we cannot remove racism from our societies. Anyone who is not combating racist policies is allowing the racism to continue. Those who are in power have a responsibility to all of their citizens. Excluding a few based on the color of their skin hurts all societies.

Reality Accepting Exercise:

Think about a time when others excluded you from an activity. How did you feel when they excluded you? Were others excluded from the activity? Did you feel they justified their reasons for excluding you? Did you keep trying to join the activity afterward? Were you excluded for obvious reasons or were they arbitrary?

Especially if you are in a marginalized group, you will know all about exclusion from other groups. Allowing yourself to understand other people's experiences with exclusionary behavior will help you understand your own experiences. Empathizing and understanding others will help you with your own life. No one lives the same life. Understanding a wide variety of other people's stories will increase your knowledge of them, yourself, and the world.

Chapter 23
Leadership and Power

Leadership

"I'm a great leader. I always have answers for everything. There is no wasting time consulting with others, looking at numbers, or twiddling my thumbs. My voice is loud, and people listen to it. When I tell someone to do something, they do it without question."

Reality Denial

"Leaders are people who try to understand what everyone they are leading needs to do their best. They listen to those they lead instead of guiding them without input. Leaders guide others. They don't demand."

Reality Acceptance

People love fantasizing about kings and queens. They continue to tell fairy tales and legends from the past as fantasy stories where dreams come true. We often romanticize these times and forget the unpleasant reality of living in a monarchy. The governments of today have problems, but they are much better than those of the past.

The monarchy fully established the class system in its traditions. If you had no power, you could complain about those in power only to others with no power. Those in power completely controlled people's behavior. Freewill was a fantasy no one exercised. Those in power had even less freewill because of the constraints of their royal obligations. You were born in your position and you stayed there. Your only choice was to uphold your position in society or accept a lower position.

More democratic systems have replaced those of the monarchy. We accepted dignity as a human right for everyone. A class system only works for those at the top. To want to be in a leadership position takes a certain amount of reality denial. Your power restrains your happiness and health. You no longer have freewill. Freewill is accepting the reality of your choices. Even fairy tales talked about living happily ever after. Today, this is more than just a fantasy. We can accept absolute power as unnecessary and harmful to society.

The leadership of today has far less power than the leadership of the past. Allowing a few people unlimited control over others rarely happens. We choose leaders to fulfill the needs of the people they are leading. If you step into an existing leadership role, they will judge you against all previous leaders. Stepping into a leadership position requires problem-solving, social skills, and sacrifice. Your time is not your own. It belongs to all the people you are leading.

A leader's primary job is solving problems. They are not good leaders if they avoid or ignore problems. The problems do not disappear, but the confidence in your leadership does. Leaders need to care for the people they are leading. Listening to them is key to understanding existing problems. Leading others means you know where you are leading them. If you are not an effective leader, those you lead will be less effective. Leaders must be able to communicate and solve problems with others. Getting help from those you are leading is just as important as helping them.

SEE MORE EXAMPLES AT:

realityacceptance.com/category/behavior/leadership/

Power

"I learned early to get power wherever I could and keep it as long as I can. If someone comes after my power, they will soon learn I will do whatever it takes to stay in power."

Reality Denial

"People who crave power are trying to fill some void in their life. The power fills in for their lack of friends, meaningful relationships, and happiness. We can use power for good in the world, but few people with power have enough of a grasp on reality to know what is good for the world. Power doesn't corrupt, it consumes."

Reality Acceptance

The history of power around the world has changed since the days of kings and queens. We limit the amount of power any one person can have. We are more educated, have more access to information, and have learned the dangers of unlimited power. Not all leaders of today have earned or deserve the power they possess. They are skilled at becoming a leader, but not necessarily at leading others.

We usually associate power with money. People who have money usually have power. People do not get into positions of power without a monetary compensation. We view people in power differently than other people. We see them as untouchable because they are most of the time. They surround themselves with people whose job is to keep others away from them. The separation from others builds a lack of real interactions with others. They become separated from other people and reality.

The more power people have, the less they can accept reality. Their actions get highly praised and criticized because they affect many lives. They worry more about their decisions than the people affected by their decisions. They cannot have genuine conversations in public because they can only speak in generalities. Their creativity, honesty, and humanity decrease the longer they are in power. They view maintaining or growing their power as more important than living a satisfying life.

Creating effective power structures is much more important than choosing leaders. The power structure must guide leaders into doing what is right for the most people. The key is creating limits. We must limit the amount, duration, and scope of the power we give people. Because we approve of one leader's use of power does not mean we can allow him or her unlimited power. Anyone with too much power is dangerous, even if we agree with them.

Reality Accepting Exercise:

Think about the best leaders you had in your life. What made them good leaders? Did you try to emulate them in your life? Did they act like traditional leaders? Were there others who disagreed with their leadership style? Are there things they did you would do differently? Did they ever have to remind you of their power over you?

Now think about the worst leader you had in your life. What made them bad leaders? Did you learn from their ineffective leadership style? Did they act like traditional leaders? Were there others who agreed with their leadership style? What would you have done differently from them? Did they ever have to remind you of their power over you?

Chapter 24
Relationships

*"I've had many relationships come
and go in my life. You might call me an
expert. I know exactly what I want in a
relationship. I haven't found it yet, but I'll
keep looking. Settling for less than perfect
is not an option for me."*

Reality Denial

*"I've had good and bad relationships
in my life. The best relationships are with
people who care about me as much as I
care about them. Expecting a relationship
to only be one way misses the point of
having relationships with other people."*

Reality Acceptance

Relationships depend on communication. If we do not
communicate effectively with others, our relationships will
suffer. We can have a mix of positive and negative
relationships with others. A positive relationship will build our
happiness and health. We will seek other positive relationships
to continue building these positive interactions and our
wellbeing. Negative relationships decrease our desire for
social interactions. This does not doom us to isolation if our
past interactions were negative. Before we can cultivate
positive relationships, we must understand how a positive
relationship works.

Reciprocation is important in any relationship. If you only take from a relationship and never give, it is a one-sided relationship. When you reciprocate to others, they will usually reciprocate back. If two people do not care for each other equally, they are not in a positive relationship. Staying in a relationship with others you do not care about is worse than leaving them. You will use them and prove yourself unworthy of the relationship. If you stay in a relationship with someone you do not trust, you will become insecure about the relationship. We should trust others until they prove undeserving of it.

If you grew up with only negative interactions in your family, you must learn how positive relationships work with others. This can be hard when you only have brief interactions with positive relationships. The interactions you saw modeled from your family may have seemed normal. The physical and mental abuse you suffered was how all families interacted as far as you knew. If you do not have positive relationships with others, you grew up in a negative household. Your initial reaction to seeing positive interactions may repel you. They will appear unnatural and fake. If your family saw you interacting this way, they would ridicule you. They saw acting positively toward others as a sign of weakness. In reality, interacting with others positively will be the most difficult and brave thing you can do.

We choose to be vulnerable with others when we are in a positive relationship with them. Without the vulnerability, we are only acquaintances. We are acquaintances with the people we work with, but being in a relationship depends on being vulnerable. Friendships develop between people when they care for each other regardless of status, power, or expectations. We choose our friends through shared interests, experiences, and caring. You will only tolerate negative friendships if you accept negative relationships. When you experience a positive relationship, you will no longer accept negative ones.

Some of the most positive and helpful relationships in people's lives are with teachers and mentors. They help you develop as a person. If you do not have positive relationships with your family or friends, a mentor can show you a positive relationship. They can be a guide for you to emulate in your other relationships. The mentor began a relationship with you because he or she wanted to help you grow as a person. Learning from the behavior of others is the best way to teach you how to behave yourself. Even if you have learned negative behaviors in the past, you can always learn positive ways to relate to others.

SEE MORE EXAMPLES AT:

realityacceptance.com/category/behavior/relationships/

Family

Reality Denial

Reality Acceptance

Your family is the first relationship that informs how you interact with others. They form a powerful impression on you as a person. They can give you your genetic traits, influence your behavior, and help you develop into adulthood. Children emulate the behavior of their family because it is the primary reality they experience. When we see non-family members acting differently to our family, they seem strange to us. If your family interacts negatively with one another, you will interact negatively with the world. Even negative relationships can help you form more positive relationships with others.

A family who all relate to one another in healthy ways is not an average family. Most societies do not value healthy relationships over such things as power, competition, and loyalty. When you live in a society that devalues healthy relationships, you do not notice their absence. This becomes more pronounced when you only see unhealthy relationships in your family. You are loyal to your family despite how unhealthy your relationship is with them. You shun positive relationships outside your family because they appear unhealthy. Positive emotions become fictional concepts only weak people talk about. Happiness becomes a mask you put on as you assume others are doing. The negative relationships in your family do not have to affect your ability to have positive relationships with others.

Seeing your parents and other family members interact with people outside your family is your first glimpse of interactions with other people. They interact differently depending on the person or group with which they interact. You learn how to interact positively with others, but you assume these interactions are fake. Being polite with strangers differs from being polite with your family. This is how you think of it, but it is not true. If you see your family as the first group of people with which you need to compete, you will see your entire life as a competition. Relationships become unhealthy competitions with other people. Your relationships will not automatically fail if you come from a family of unhealthy relationships, but you will need to find examples of healthy relationships outside your family.

Instead of competing with your family, you can study them. Do not tell them you are studying them, but you can use how they relate to you and others to judge positive and negative interactions. You are like a scientist studying the behavior of animals in nature. If they are unhappy most of the time, observe what behaviors correspond to their negative mood. Use this information to inform how you relate to others.

When I was a child, I noticed how frustrated my dad would get when he could not figure out how to put something together. He would only read the manual if his frustration level reached a certain point. I learned not only to read manuals, but how to avoid frustration.

Learning healthy relationships is a matter of accepting what a healthy relationship looks like. Healthy relationships do not appear in the entertainment, competitions, or other heightened views of reality we interact with regularly. The traditions and ceremonies we learned as kids seemed like positive interactions, but are they? It shocks most people when they hear or see themselves in a recording. If I see myself in the reflection of a window, I want to look away because the reality is shocking. We pose for pictures to avoid seeing the reality of what we normally look like. The problem is not what we look like in our natural states, but accepting ourselves in our natural states.

Reality shows must heighten interactions in them because most reality is boring. We want our interactions with others as exaggerated as these shows. We do not find yelling and exaggerated gestures in most conversations with people we care about. You can always tell who is unaware they are on a hidden camera show by their low-key reactions. Actors in movies are usually not acting naturally because that would make boring movies. Exaggerating anything beyond a natural amount is unnatural. People told me most of my life that I was too calm. I now realize this was mainly because of my lack of exaggerated reactions to others. This is a common reaction to people with autism. They are speaking naturally, but it is not the usual exaggerated style most people expect.

The only healthy relationships are those in which all involved care equally for one another. It is the reality of love, but not what we call love. Few times in our lives are we surrounded by people who care about us as much as we care about them. We call our family members loved ones, but do not care equally about them. If we treat each other equally, we would be more concerned about the emotional reasons behind negative behavior than the behavior itself. Teenagers who say they hate their parents are using extreme language to express their emotions. If teenagers hated their parents, they would not care about expressing their emotions to them. I would worry more about an unemotional teenager than an emotional one.

Accepting the reality of your family is about accepting the reality of who they are as people. We focus only on either the positive or negative traits of our family and ignore the less extreme traits. These less extreme traits make up who they are most of the time. Life is not just things you hate or things you love. Sometimes caring about your family lets them make mistakes. A sizable family can have healthy relationships with one another, but they are difficult. Just as a small company can give more individual attention to their employees, a sizable family has a limited amount of time to care individually for one another. If you can describe each of your family members with one or two words, you do not know them well. We do not choose most of our family, but we can choose how we relate to them.

Friendships

Reality Denial

Reality Acceptance

Your friends are people you are in a relationship with by choice, unlike your relationship with your family. Childhood friendships can develop into adult friendships, but they must change over time because people change throughout their lives. They require constant reinforcement because there is no inherent expectation of the relationship. You will both change separately without your relationship changing if you spend time apart. I am closer with friends I kept in touch with than my best friends with which I lost touch. It is essential to maintain your friendships to keep up with their changing lives. Valuing your friendships will value your happiness and health.

If you need your friends for more than emotional support, they are not your friends. Needing your friends to validate you as a person will lead to you using them. Friends are not those who spiral into depression with you, they prevent you from becoming depressed. They help you solve problems for yourself instead of solving them for you. Not having friends will lead to unhealthy relationships throughout your life. When I was early in my teen years, I found myself with no close friends. This was partially because they separated me from my friends when I changed schools, but also because I was not good at forming friendships. I spiraled into depression and contemplated suicide. Luckily, I did not carry out these thoughts. Having even one valued friendship would have prevented my severe depression.

Friendship requires an equal level of caring for one another. If the relationship is not equal, it is not a friendship. Your parents cannot be your friends until you are both adults. A teacher is not your friend until she is no longer your teacher. A friendship will not last if one person feels they are an unequal partner. Friendships based on anything other than caring for one another are not valuable friendships. If we never convert strangers into friends, we will live our lives surrounded by strangers. Dealing with strangers is inherently unequal because you either do not know how they view you or you know they view you as unequal to them. A friendship is a balanced relationship that helps keep you mentally healthy throughout your life.

When I married my wife, I married my best friend. We were friends before we started a romantic relationship. I would recommend this to anyone who is thinking about getting married. This may sound obvious to you, but it is not obvious to everyone. Friendship should lead to dating and marriage. If you skip being friends and living together, your marriage has less of a chance of working. Many religions discourage this practice at the detriment of marriages everywhere. A divorce is not a failure of the marriage, it is a failure of a friendship that did not develop and grow. My wife and I disagree, but our friendship always wins out.

People who matter to you are different from people you care about. The server at your favorite restaurant matters to you, but he is not your friend. Genuine friendships will help you live a happier and longer life. Healthy family relationships will lead to you developing healthy friendships. Valuing these friendships is important for valuing yourself as a person. A balanced friendship will help you deal with problems, handle hardship, and add to the quality of your life. Having quality friends is about being a quality friend yourself. This does not mean you behave the same as your friends. It only means you care about them as much as they care about you.

SEE MORE EXAMPLES AT:

realityacceptance.com/category/behavior/friendships/

Reality Accepting Exercise:

Think about your closest relationships you value the most in your life. Why do they mean so much to you? Do you feel you could tell them anything? Are your closest relationships with your family or friends? Do you consider your family as friends? What are the major differences between people you are close with and people you are not? Are your closest relationships like you or not like you?

Relating to other people is something we do throughout our lives. Close relationships are rare and special. Examining your close relationships is one of the best ways to examine yourself. How you relate to your closest friends should be how you relate to everyone. As you go through your day, think of everyone as potential close friends.

Chapter 25
Cultures and Societies

Cultures

"I don't feel a part of any culture. Cultures have no influence on me and I don't care about other people's cultures. I just follow whatever is popular, and that is my culture."

Reality Denial

"There are many different cultures that have influenced me in my life. No single culture dominates who I am as a person. I always welcome discovering new cultures to give me a wider view of the world."

Reality Acceptance

The cultures that influence us are the groups of people we relate to beyond our family, friends, and teachers. They influence our interactions with others and help form us as people. They provide a series of unwritten rules that let us know what appropriate behavior in our local area is. Your family's acceptance of the culture will influence your attitude toward it. If the dominant culture rejects your family, the culture will reject you. You can distance yourself from your family for acceptance into the culture, but that will deny you as a person and your past. If you do not know why this will damage you, you need to start this book over from the beginning.

We do not plan cultural communities. We develop them through many influences and factors that are not conscious within the community. A community of humans is much more complex than a colony of ants. The ants seem to act with one mind because they are simple organisms whose actions are instinctual. You will have less freedom in a culture with less diversity. The leaders of the culture act as the parents for those in it. Those leaders have far less interest in you as an individual than your parents. The culture develops to fulfill the needs of the leaders because they are directing its growth. Anyone who does not adhere to these needs will have difficulty in the culture. Cultures are as complex as the individuals who make them up.

There are multiple cultures that influence us. Cultures can comprise a shared location, ethnicity, economic group, interests, or many other factors. You can grow up in one culture and add several other cultures throughout your life. The more cultures that influence you, the more diverse cultures you will join. When you experience a new culture, you can better understand the cultures that have influenced you. Each culture will have its advantages and disadvantages. One culture will allow you more freedom, but at the expense of your safety. Another will give you stability, but at the expense of your education. Experiencing multiple cultures throughout your life will allow you to grow as a person.

Cultures that do not accept reality will lead to individuals who deny reality. Cultures centered on myths, segregation, isolation, hatred, or any other reality denying activities will lead to unhappy and unhealthy members. The culture will punish members who accept realities they reject. The more simplistic the realities a culture rejects, the unhealthier the culture will grow and develop. Cultures that do not grow and change will find their members dwindling as generations grow out of the outdated values.

The cultures in your life will influence you, whether they embrace or reject you. No one should accept one culture at the expense of all others. Cultures influence you, but you do not represent them. I am a member of male culture, but I reject most of its values. The cultures influential to you should vary as much as the knowledge you collect throughout your life. Being multicultural will allow you to grow and develop as a person. Isolating yourself from cultures you do not understand will isolate you from most other cultures. Understanding other cultures is an exciting and necessary part of your growth as a person.

Societies

*"We're so fractured in society today
it's not even funny. I was talking to this
lady, and she was barely speaking English.
Nothing she said made sense to me. I told
her, 'Why don't you go back to your
society that speaks your language?' She
just walked away from me as if I said
something rude, like she would understand
if I did."*

Reality Denial

*"If you live in an area where several
different cultures exist, each of the cultures
is a part of the society. Unfortunately, the
rules of the society usually only come from
a few of the cultures. To have a society
that works well together, we must all take
part in it."*

Reality Acceptance

Societies comprise many cultures. One culture may dominate, but it is not representative of most of the cultures in the society. All members of the society rarely choose the leaders of the society. Cultures that value power dominate most societies. The only distinguishing factor among all members of a society is location. People refer to the values of a society, but it is only the values of the dominant culture. Individuals vary in any society just as the biological life varies in an ecosystem. The leaders and members of a society must embrace change and diversity for a society to grow and thrive.

Accepting the diversity of all members will lead to a healthy society.

A cohesive society requires compromise by all of its members. No culture can get everything they desire without compromising what other cultures desire. A society representing more diverse voices will make a healthier society. Even in a totalitarian society, the dominant culture must make compromises to prevent revolt by the dominated citizens. In a more democratic society, compromise is key to maintaining the democracy for the greatest number of people. No single culture should get too much or too little power. If unrest exists in a society, the society will destroy itself or another society will destroy it. Compromise allows a society to maintain a healthy balance of power.

The borders between different societies can be physical or emotional. Leaders can use fear and false promises to manipulate their citizens. A society connected by lies will eventually stop believing the lies. It may take generations before change happens, but a society's people will not remain powerless forever. We have claimed all the areas of the world and split them up into different societies. You can stay in the society you are in or join another one. Knowledge of other societies is available to most people. Even if the leaders are lying to its citizens, factual information will get past the borders. You are not completely blind to what other societies can offer you. Fear keeps most people in a society where they have no power. Borders become obstacles to your happiness and health you must overcome.

Most societies have rules that apply to all of their citizens. Those in power may ignore these rules, but they know the rules they are breaking. These rules can be in the form of laws, expected behaviors, or implied expectations of the society members. Breaking the rules can get you ostracized, punished, or killed. When only a few members of a society create these rules, they become mocked, ignored, or rebelled against. These rules will only last as long as those members remain in power. The rules of a healthy society will form a balanced compromise of acceptable behavior by all of its citizens.

Most people recognize the diversity within their own society, but view other societies as less diverse. Societies go well beyond their borders. It is rare to find a society made up of only generations of past citizens. Societies hostile to diversity are becoming more of a rarity. Learning about other societies can be the most interesting and exciting knowledge you receive. Restricting yourself to only understanding the society in which you live will lead to unhealthy relationships with other societies. Societies are neither negative nor positive. The only commonality among all the citizens in a society is living in the same location. Only by experiencing another society directly or from a member of that society can we understand our own.

SEE MORE EXAMPLES AT:

realityacceptance.com/category/behavior/societies/

Individuality in Societies

*"I am a rule follower and a group
joiner. I don't know why other people
don't just shut up and go along with the
program. If everyone does something one
way, why would I do it differently?"*

Reality Denial

*"I rarely go along with what most
people do. If you want me not to do
something, just tell me that everyone's
doing it."*

Reality Acceptance

A tolerance for other people and their behaviors is important
to accepting others. We need to be tolerant of unfamiliar
behaviors and thinking, especially when dealing with people
from other cultures. We cannot judge others until we
understand them. Intolerant people will conflict with
unfamiliar individuals who do not fit in to the dominant
culture. We discourage individuality within many societies. If
too many people act as individuals, a collectivist society will
fracture. We must balance individualism and collectivism if
we are to work together as a society.

When I was young, I was an individualist. I prided myself
on doing things my way. I did not accept peer pressure or help
from others unless it coincided with my ways of doing things.
This was mainly because I was a shy kid. As I got older, I
have added more collectivist thinking to my view of other
people. I now care about others as much as I care about

myself. My individuality should not impede the needs of others. I am a creative individualist and a caring collectivist.

Allowing people to act as individuals helps a society advance in technology, creativity, and free expression. Individuality has given us alternative forms of art, entertainment, and science. Without individuality, life would cease to be interesting. Not that individualism is always good for society. Isolating yourself and only doing things your own way can separate you from both the rules and the help of society. You will need to follow the rules and accept help from society to create something unique. It is more inventive to create something within limits than creating something with no limits.

Politics

"I don't know why movies and TV shows have to feature transgender and gay characters in them. Why do they have to make everything political? They're just shoving their gay agenda and political correctness in our face."

Reality Denial

"We developed politics to give a voice to the people through representatives who represent the voice of those people. That is how it works in the ideal. Unfortunately, that ideal has developed into a competition between two opposing teams. I hope politicians can see they represent everyone, not just the ones who voted for them."

Reality Acceptance

Societies have developed politics to balance the needs of all the people within them. It was a better system than a dictatorship for everyone except the dictators. Different societies developed their governments to ensure societies could cooperate and not descend into chaos. Societies not equally balancing the wants of its leaders and citizens died out. The Roman Empire is an example of one such society. Modern societies accept that all its members must compromise to work effectively together, but not all of them agree on who is a member of their society.

The photographer for my high school graduation photo told me I should run for political office. This insulted me because I saw politics as a miserable job I would not wish on anyone. Was she assuming I had no skills other than smiling and being polite to people? I had a pleasant smile and people rarely knew what I really thought of them, but that was no reason to wish me a miserable life. I know her words were not malicious. She was merely expressing a long-standing belief of many people. Most politicians only have power to maintain the status quo, and that did not appeal to me.

Current political systems are better than historical ones, but they are not perfect. Most of the problems are carryovers from the past. Policies still exist that allow special interest groups, people with wealth and power, and large corporations to exert more control over the political system than most of the people affected by them. This happens because our focus is on political ads, news, ideologies, race, sexual orientation, debates, and other irrelevant factors. Choosing qualified candidates who can solve problems is the only consideration relevant to their jobs.

The best politician is one who absorbs all sides of an issue and supports the idea that accomplishes the best outcome for the most people. Politicians have developed the skill of pandering to those who elected them or will do so. The only qualification for most candidates is to entertain the most people. Politicians have taken over for the clowns of the past. Someday, politicians will sink to the level of being too creepy to vote for as clowns have become too creepy to entertain. Quality politicians must balance their problem solving and entertainment skills.

Vote for policies, not people. When I hear people say, "I am voting for the candidate I can have a beer with," I cringe. We are not voting for politicians just so we can hang out with them and be friends. Most of the politicians I have voted for were people I did not want to be friends with. I voted for them to make the best decisions for the most people, and their stances on policies are the best sign of that. Some people will say that always voting for one party is wrong. This would be true if most political races had over two parties running. I have only voted for Democrats because I do not agree with most of the policies of Republicans. I would choose a more moderate candidate if I could, but they do not exist in most elections.

Most political parties only focus on the extremes of issues. Are you for or against this issue? If you express a nuanced thought about an issue, people will ignore you for a more extreme politician. Politicians have platforms that read like a list of likes and dislikes. I do not care if you claim human rights as important to you. What policies are you proposing to ensure we value the human rights of others under your leadership? Many politicians focus on small and unimportant issues to distract from larger issues they cannot easily solve. These insignificant issues are many times the only problems politicians can hope to fix. Promising the world to voters is unrealistic, but often done.

Voters often vote against candidates rather than voting for them. They are voting "No" on candidates and issues by voting "Yes" for other candidates and issues. They make one candidate out to be the hero because they already think of the other candidates as villains. Many people see this as a reason to not vote. If no politician is talking about issues affecting you, why should you? Most times, you would be better off putting your energy toward creating change outside of politics. We should view voting as hiring the candidates for a job we want them to do. Politicians who spend years in politics only concentrate on their reelection. We need to vote for new and more qualified politicians to solve problems and affect change.

In many countries, we choose our leaders from a conservative or liberal candidate. It is a choice between wanting change and keeping the status quo. These are rarely the politicians who will balance the needs of the most people. Knowledge of social issues, economics, and negotiation will create the best compromises among citizens, businesses, and social institutions. Things that should be are not the reality of most situations. My advice to anyone who reads this is to avoid social media, political debates, political ads, and anything not informing you how well a candidate can solve problems. Problems come in all shapes and sizes. Choose candidates who are logical and accept the realities of issues. They will be the best problem solvers.

People sometimes say, "I don't mean to be political, but…" This means they are trying not to express an opinion about politics. You can talk about politics without expressing an opinion about it. Mentioning politicians' actions is not expressing an opinion about them or politics. Many people find it difficult to talk about politics without expressing a political opinion. We see political parties like we see sports teams. We express our opinions about our "team" through our votes. Political opinions divide us in conversations, but the political process unites us through our common issues.

Being politically correct has little to do with politics. Its origins come from politicians avoiding sensitive topics to avoid offending voters. Today, people use it as a reason not to care about others. Caring about others comes from caring about yourself. People who do not care about themselves do not care about others. We treat others well because there is no reason to mistreat them. Talking negatively about other people you do not know is expressing an opinion about something you do not understand. We need less ignorant opinions about politics and more knowledge in the world.

SEE MORE EXAMPLES AT:

realityacceptance.com/category/behavior/politics/

Reality Accepting Exercise:

Think about how many cultures have influenced you throughout your life. They can be your family, friends, neighbors, co-workers, classmates, the area where you grew up, or other people who influenced you. Did the number of cultural influences increase as you aged? Was there a main cultural influence? Are there cultural influences you chose not to accept? Were you influenced more by family or external cultures? Are your friends from similar cultures or different ones?

Our cultures influence who we are and how we live our lives. Some cultures value the people in them, and others value the traditions of the culture more. We should never consider ourselves only part of one culture. It usually means you will never get to know people from other cultures. Diversity is important for understanding other people. The cultures who shelter their members from other cultures separate themselves from the world at large. This has both good and bad consequences.

Part 6
Reality Accepted

Chapter 26
The Reality of Accepting Reality

This last section of the book deals with issues you may deal with once you have the skills to accept reality. As stated at the beginning of the book, I did not teach you about reality. I taught you the skills of recognizing reality when we can know it. You will still find aspects of life with no simple answers. Accepting what we cannot know is as important as accepting what we can. As I accepted more reality in my life, I found specific issues coming up when dealing with other people. You have accepted reality, but most people have not. I have come up with some strategies for dealing with reality in a reality denying world.

You may feel defensive about your Reality Acceptance. Everyone around you is denying realities you now cannot ignore. Traditions and habits you previously took part in will seem illogical and a waste of time. You do not have to spread the word of Reality Acceptance, nor should you. People will resent you pointing out the reality they are ignoring. You can point out realities to others, but let them decide if they want to accept them. Many people will reject realities that force them to see the world differently. Most people fear change. You do not have to convince them to accept reality in one conversation. Help them with problems they are dealing with without telling them about realities they are ignoring.

How do you deal with your current life when you used to hate the person you are? When I went through my reality accepting journey, I had to convince my wife I was a changed person from the one she married. The things that made me anxious or angry in the past seemed trivial now. I could handle any problem because I viewed them realistically. My old self was a reality denying version of me. I feel sorry for him because I know he was miserable much of the time. I embraced the logical thinking I always had in the back of my mind and implemented it in my life. If being logical is wrong, I don't want to be right!

Part of accepting reality is knowing what reality is important to your happiness and health. Sometimes, you need a break from reality overload. There is much suffering and tragedy that happens every minute of every day around the world. If you spend your time worrying about these things, you are not helping other people to change their circumstances. To change the world, you need to experience it directly. You cannot watch negative events happening far away and help change them. Even if you are experiencing a negative event, you can only affect change if it is realistically possible. I will not go to an event with which I strongly disagree because it will only lead to negative results.

You cannot accept reality by removing yourself from it. The reality of a situation does not go away when you do. Reality is motionless unless someone or something affects it. Reading this book has hopefully started you thinking about all the realities most people ignore. If you think something will never change, you are missing the incremental changes happening every day. Major changes happen rarely, but they happen. You may think minor changes will not affect your life overall, but those changes add up. Understanding reality is the first step to solving problems, but it is not the only step. We must use our direct knowledge of reality to change it for the better.

One hurdle in accepting reality is accepting smaller realities and ignoring larger ones. You yell at someone because they are mistreating another person, but you ignore you are making the situation worse. We can only change negative behavior with the cooperation of the person behaving negatively. We must handle societal and cultural problems from the top down. If abuse is prevalent in a culture, you cannot stop every abuser individually. You must understand the cultural problems causing the prevalence of the abuse. Abuse is a problem in many cultures, but there are varied and complex reasons we must understand. Focusing on a single abuser ignores the larger issue.

Some people focus on solving minor problems to avoid solving major ones. We accept that we have a problem with our health, but we only resolve to drink more water during the day. Drinking more water is good, but it ignores the food we eat, our lack of exercise, and our mental health. Minor changes can lead to more changes, but minor changes should not be at the expense of major changes. We are wasting much of our time on minor problems. If we focus more on major problems, we will resolve most of the minor problems. Once you have resolved the major problems for yourself, you can help others with their problems. We need to help them solve major problems first, and they will solve their minor problems on their own.

Many people consider entertainment to be frivolous and unnecessary to their happiness and health. We need relief from reality in the form of fictional realities. Experiencing someone else's story is the best way to get to know them. We cannot live their life, but we can experience life from their perspective. Most of us cannot afford to travel to other people to experience their stories, but we can hear, read, and view their stories as entertainment. Stories that elicit diverse emotional responses provide the most well-rounded entertainment. Some people complain about stories with happy endings, but I find positive change at the story's end to be far more entertaining than negative endings. Stories are about resolving fictional problems, not presenting unresolved problems. Entertainment should relieve us from negative realities, not focus on unresolved problems.

It may concern you that Reality Acceptance will hamper your ability to fantasize or dream. Examining reality might not allow you to see anything beyond what you know is real. I can tell you that my imagination is greater now than it has ever been. I have been a fan of fantasy stories my entire life and still am. There is a reality to our fantasies and dreams, allowing us to experience things we cannot experience in our actual life. Our imaginations allow us to create stories in which our dreams come true. The best part about imagining a dream coming true is being able to change the story to suit newer dreams.

The biggest lesson I hope you have learned from this book is solving problems. You can think of yourself as a reality detective. The more reality you accept, the better you can solve problems. Complex problems involve more factors and will take longer to solve. We can only solve minor problems quickly. The more minor problems you solve, the more confident you will feel about solving major ones. At the

end of this book, I present ideas for how we can solve some of
our major problems around the world with Reality
Acceptance. The solutions involve others accepting the reality
of situations and their part in them. I am fully aware I am
asking for an unrealistic acceptance of reality on a major scale.
I accept I am a dreamer, but I am not the only one.

The Reality of Reality Acceptance

Reality Acceptance is a habit that gets better the more
experience you have with it. Like any habit, it takes time to
allow yourself to see the realities of any situation instead of
the assumptions, beliefs, and negative emotions you have
lived with for years. It is only the first step in solving any
problem, crisis, or situation. You will need to see things from
other points of view and give everyone the benefit of the
doubt. This will not be easy when people are openly hostile to
you. They are only hostile to what you represent in their mind.
You can still care about them, even if they are yelling at you.

Even when you accept reality more, you will deny reality
you do not understand. When you do this, it is good to confess
your ignorance to yourself. Sometimes we need to remind
ourselves of our ignorance. When you notice it, acknowledge
it, and learn from it. People deny reality more out of habit than
feeling hostility toward some part of reality. We accept the
realities we commonly deal with, but deny realities with which
we have little experience. Reality denial comes from our
beliefs. Beliefs are temporary impressions of the world.
Negative emotions come from beliefs, and positive emotions
come from knowledge. Accepting positive emotions is about
accepting reality.

Sometimes we need to accept that other people do not accept reality. This may seem easy in a world that does not accept reality most of the time. As you will discover, it is overwhelming when you realize the amount of reality people ignore, deny, or do not think about. I had a list of all the reality denial I saw daily, but I had to stop adding to it because it was endless. People deny realities they fear, or wish were not true. The best you can do for them is stay out of their way or help them if you can. You cannot help most people, but that does not have to ruin your day. The most we can do is make the world a better place for ourselves and people who will accept reality.

You will become a positive barrier to other people when you stop rushing your way through your day. A positive barrier is something preventing them from denying reality. Few people rush through life for genuine reasons. All you need to do is treat them better than they treat themselves. They all have unresolved issues in their lives. Learn from them and do not run from your own issues. If you find yourself in a hurry, slow down and deal with the problem that is pushing you into being in a hurry. Accepting reality does not mean only having simple problems. It is about finding out all you can about the problem so you can start forming plans for working on it. The problem is usually not as difficult to solve as you think.

Making decisions is more difficult when you feel resistance toward your choices. If you only include a few factors in a decision, you will see fewer choices. Never create fixed rules while deciding on something. Think of the issue in as many ways as you can. Do not discount any factors you consider deal breakers. Brainstorming is not about finding solutions; it is about gathering information. It takes time to gather information and think about all the factors involved in making complex life decisions. If you think there are only a few choices involved, you need to gather more information and factors.

Reality Accepting Exercise:

Think about the realities I have talked about in this book. Of all of them, what realities did you have the toughest time with? Are you still having a tough time accepting them fully? Are the realities personal or do they involve other people? Have you always had problems with these realities or are they recent problems? Are they simple or complex realities?

Hopefully, you realize by the last section of this book that there are no simple realities. That last question is a trap. Do not fall for it. The hardest realities to deal with involve conflicts in our perception of reality. People who deny realities you care about are the hardest to deal with. It is easy to dismiss strangers when their reality denial is extreme, but it can be heartbreaking when you know the harm people you care about are doing to themselves. As I mentioned earlier in the book, work on helping them and not their reality denial.

Chapter 27

Reality Overload

Reality overload can cause stress, anxiety, health problems, social problems, and a general negativity to your life. Usually, reality is not the problem. The problem exists when we overload ourselves with other people's perceptions of reality or their denial of reality. As long as you do not accept the stress and anxiety of others, they will bother you less. If you accept reality as either relevant or irrelevant to your life, you can filter out the reality overload. This will be easier for some people than others.

I heard someone say they had to "hack up a fur ball of stress" once. Being a cat person, I really liked that phrase. Unfortunately, humans cannot hack up fur balls of stress to relieve their stress. The closest we can come is decreasing stressful situations in our lives. External factors can cause stress, but it is the internal acceptance of these factors that cause the stress on our bodies. People handle problems differently. We can stress out by overloading ourselves with factors involved in a problem. When we break the problem down into manageable steps, we can solve it without the stress.

As a shy child, I had severe anxiety problems. I can still remember many of the anxious experiences from my childhood. Looking back, I can now pinpoint why I was anxious and what I could have done to relieve or avoid the anxious situations. I rarely get anxious today because I understand the reality behind the anxiety. I was anxious about minor problems. External forces did not cause my anxieties. They came from internal perceptions, fears, and misconceptions. My vivid imagination worked against my perception of reality. I imagined everyone was looking at me, seeing every mistake I made, and would never want to be friends with me. Only a few kids were looking at me, I had processing issues leading to errors in judgment, and my anxieties made it hard to make friends. Everyone has anxiety, but only people who accept their anxiety can deal with it.

Some people cannot look away from a car crash. Days after they see the crash, the world becomes filled with car crashes. The world is not more dangerous, but they perceive it that way because of their emotions about the recent car crash. Focusing only on the negative aspects of reality will lead to a negative view of the world. The more you focus only on negative realities, the more negative your perceptions of reality will be. Forcing yourself to notice positive things will draw your attention away from negative ones.

Some reality can seem overwhelming if you do not understand it. Accepting reality does not mean you understand all of reality. Humanity may never understand some realities. You only need to understand the reality relevant to your life. People can find themselves with an excess of information without the knowledge of how to process it. If something seems overwhelming, search for information that simplifies the subject. When you understand the general reality of the subject, you can move on to more complex understandings.

Sometimes we do things based on habits or traditions rather than what is actually relevant to our lives. We stress about realities that have no real baring on us. Questioning the relevance of realities will help you avoid stressing over irrelevant ones. Examining and evaluating them becomes more difficult the longer we spend without questioning them.

The more realities you question, the better you can understand them and evaluate their relevance to you.

Unavoidable Realities

We cannot avoid some realities. Not dealing with them will only make them worse. We cannot hide from some realities or their causes. Death, hurricanes, tsunamis, and cancer are situations you cannot avoid when you experience them. If you do not take them seriously, you will wish you had. They are realities you cannot change because they are unchangeable. They are instant unpleasant facts we cannot undo. Accepting the reality of the problems will not solve the problems they cause. You can only mitigate their effects. Reality is controlling you more than you can control it.

I am writing this during the pandemic of 2020. It is definitely an unavoidable reality on a global scale. People can deny the seriousness of it, but they cannot avoid dealing with the effects of it in their daily lives. Some people see it as a prison sentence and others accept the limits it places on them. How you view it is completely up to you. If you believe it has impeded your rights, you will downplay the safety concerns. If your family gets sick, you cannot avoid how your actions affect them. The only difference is how much you care about your family versus other people. The reality for everyone was the same.

An undeniable reality is one you cannot ignore. It creates barriers you cannot deny unless you ignore major realities. You will not be running through the park if you break your leg. If you do not accept this barrier, you cannot go beyond it. You can severely damage your health if you ignore the reality of the barrier. Barriers are merely the limits we must deal with in our lives. You can deny you are obese until you can no longer walk out of your house. It is not a reality preventing you from living your life, but it will definitely present you with challenges.

The more marginalized groups people are in, the more unavoidable realities they will face in their lives. Marginalized groups can include women, people of color, people in the LGBTQ community, young people, older adults, neurodivergent people, the poor, and any group the dominant society has disadvantaged for being who they are. The disadvantages can increase the more groups you are in. Your ability to accept reality is a given, but you may still deny reality to protect yourself. People in multiple marginalized groups can feel empowered, ashamed, or somewhere in between about who they are. Hopefully, these groups will become accepted the more people accept reality.

The barriers or limits in our lives are necessary and can help us. A cabinet preventing a child from getting dangerous chemicals could save the child's life. We need unavoidable barriers to limit our ability to harm ourselves or other people. They impede the progress of reality denial by presenting truths we cannot ignore. Science has advanced as far as it has because scientists have accepted the laws of physics. We have proven the limits of gravity on earth. Birds can fly because they follow the laws of physics, while humans cannot because of our physical limitations. We have overcome those limitations using our ingenuity, but the limitations still exist to the unaided human body.

Some unavoidable realities happen because of circumstances beyond our control. If you have a handicap, you cannot avoid your need for help from others. People trapped in a burning building will need help from firefighters to get out. The help is available, but some people will damage their health to avoid asking others for it. You can avoid these realities, but you will pay for the consequences. The final unavoidable consequence may be death. We should accept unavoidable realities so we can handle our limitations to the best of our ability.

Live Events

Live events are not inherently positive or negative. Most people think only of the positive aspects of them. We see a band we like at a concert, hangout with friends at a party, or watch our favorite team at a stadium. There are inherently negative events such as mass shootings, violent protests, and other tragic events, but they are rare. I never enjoyed live events, mainly because of my sensory overload issues. After I fully accepted the realities of live events, they became even less appealing. You may feel similarly about live events when you experience them after reading this book. I will point out that recognizing the negative aspects of some live events does not prevent you from enjoying other live events.

The first thing you should do when going to a live event is accept the realities inherent in it. Depending on the event, there are experiences you must tolerate. If you go to a concert, you will experience enormous crowds, loud noises, inappropriate behavior, and technical errors. Accepting these things as probable will lead to a more pleasant experience. If you expect only positive experiences, you will always be disappointed. Accept that people will behave inappropriately, the show will have errors, and you will need to protect your ears to avoid hearing damage. Each event will have different inherent realities. If you are going to an event with which you have no experience, find out the realities of the event before you go.

A live event involving competition will involve several negative probabilities to accept. The experience will include overcrowding, lines, fighting, yelling, loud noises, and consumption of alcohol. Alcohol may prevent some people from remembering these experiences, but they are still likely to happen. The crowd's emotions will be high and a group mentality may take them over. If you are with the crowd, you may think of them as coming together in solidarity. If you are against the crowd, you will experience their negativity. A group does not think as one, but they can act as one. They will see you not as a person, but as a part of the competition. Competition is inherently negative, but a live event involving competition requires acceptance of an overwhelming amount of negative realities.

News on the Internet and television may not seem like a live event, but many times they are. Even videos played after they recorded the event were live. The news prides itself on presenting the latest information in an event. They are duty bound to report the news people care about. Presenting live news is a business that needs viewers and listeners to make money. As with any other live event, they depend on making money because it costs money to present the event. The news makes money through advertisers, ratings, and developing a following. People want to be on the news so they can tell their family and friends they were on the news. If people do not want to be on the news, they will definitely find themselves on the news.

Unlike other live events, live news has no guarantee of applying to everyone watching it. Live news must be so general that it is the least informative form of news. Stories must be emotionally interesting to keep the audience interested. Watching or listening to live news will only elicit an emotional response or boredom. They present information people want to know as a debatable issue. News outlets have lost money by reporting improper or untrue information. This has led to only reporting simple and easily debatable stories irrelevant to most people. My only suggestion for live news is to avoid it when you can.

We must consider the dangerous realities in some live events such as protests, rallies, and demonstrations. We must weigh the risks against the benefits. If you feel strongly about something, you may regret not attending the event. If you put your safety at risk, you may hinder your ability to take part in future events. We should consider each event individually with a realistic view toward the outcomes. If the safety concerns outweigh the benefits, you would be better off somewhere else.

Reality Relevance

Not all reality applies to everyone. We are better off ignoring some realities. Any event affecting your life or the people you know should take precedence over irrelevant events. Ignoring these events does not make them irrelevant to others, but their affect is only relevant to you through other people. Ignorance is not bliss; it is realistic. Humans love to multitask, but we do not do it well. We can only focus on one event or issue at a time. If you are rushing to get your kids to school, only focus on relevant information that gets them to school efficiently and safely. Devoting your attention to only relevant information will allow you to solve problems in a more focused way.

The world is full of reality. If we focused on all of it, we would become overloaded. We fill our days with sleeping, eating, working, and taking care of our basic human needs. We have a limited amount of time and energy to take in the reality beyond what applies to us. It seems appealing to go to one source of information about the world, but this is relying on it alone to choose what information applies to you. The best you can do is gather information from multiple sources of varied points of view. Just like avoiding negative people, avoid sources who only present information in negative ways. Information is not always positive, but the way others present it should be free of hate and other negative emotions.

We can only examine reality as snapshots of time and will never really understand it completely. If we try to examine both relevant and irrelevant realities, the irrelevant realities will distract us from relevant ones. Without a relevant external source of information, we cannot know what realities to accept. We will accept realities relevant to other people, but not ourselves. When I was younger, I noticed many people in my family were alcoholics. This information was accurate, but not relevant to me. I proved in high school I could stop eating sugar when I noticed the negative health effects. My relatives had addictive personalities because they ignored the traumas that were making them susceptible to addictions, not because of our common genes. Accepting relevant realities could have saved them from seeing alcoholism as being inevitable as I did. They could have fixed their underlying problems instead of focusing on irrelevant realities.

Reality Accepting Exercise:

Think of a time when you confronted several unavoidable realities at once. Whether you were at a live event, had several tragedies happen at once, or they put you in a situation in which there was too much happening around you. How did you handle the situation? Were there things you could have done to prevent the overload? Did you learn how to prevent future overloading situations? Did you actively do breathing or other exercises to calm yourself down? If the overwhelming situation happened today, would you react differently?

Dealing with sensory overload can be difficult when the situation is new to you. If you grew up in a large city, had a large family, and had days filled with chaotic events, you may never find yourself overwhelmed by life. You have developed coping mechanisms to deal with the overload. If your days are much calmer, you will need to develop ways of dealing with this overload. This can mean preventing the overload, dealing with it, or learning from it. Understanding your reaction to it will help you deal with it.

Chapter 28
Reality Relief

Sometimes you need a distraction from reality to handle anxiety, stress, or other negative emotions. From living in an over-crowded world to 24-hour news cycles, we are all inundated with stressful realities. People who have money and power can insulate themselves from reality, but most people cannot. We need relief from reality to maintain our health. Entertainment and relaxation can help relieve the negative effects of reality overload. Failing to relieve ourselves from the overload will lead to an unhappy and unhealthy life.

Getting enough sleep and relaxation are some of the best ways to relieve stress. If you find yourself with a break from stressful situations, do not move on to other stressful situations. Take the time to relieve stress so you can give your mind and body a chance to recuperate. Mindfulness is a practice helping many people. Most people only think of meditation when they hear the term, but there are many other mindful practices. With it, you are conscious of your body, mind, and environment. I have always struggled with sleep and stress. Meditation never seemed to work for me, but other mindful practices did. I still struggle with them, but far less frequently. Finding a mindful practice that works for you can help you get better sleep and have less stress.

Life is entertaining if you take the time to notice it. There is every genre and type of entertainment for people to escape from reality. If entertainment stresses you out, it is not entertaining. Humans developed entertainment to relieve themselves from uninteresting or negative realities. Whether it is a comedy or drama, we entertain ourselves by seeing another version of reality from our own. Some people devote most of their lives to entertaining others. Consuming and creating entertainment can help you understand and accept reality. A happier and healthier life is just around the corner.

When you accept more reality in your life, you will realize there are more positive aspects to it than negative. The chief source of negativity will come from others who do not accept reality. You can suggest they read this book, but they will not. Pointing out the positive aspects of reality is an effective strategy for getting them to see more positivity for themselves. Make sure they consider it a positive thing. Pointing things out they have negative associations with will push them further away from you and reality. When I see others who do not accept reality, I either laugh or feel sorry for them. I want others to see the positive reality in the world that I see.

We can use therapy to help us accept realities we cannot see for ourselves. Once we see the realities for ourselves, we can use this knowledge to access problems in our lives and fix them. You can do this with a therapist or on your own. Sometimes we are not the authorities on ourselves we think we are. An outside perspective can strip away the experiences, beliefs, and perceptions preventing us from seeing who we really are. If we resist the help we are getting, we are resisting the realities we fear. Someone examining us can be a vulnerable experience. If you are not vulnerable, therapy will not help you.

Stories

Stories are a way of examining other people's lives. The closest you can get to living life in someone else's shoes is hearing their story. Before we had written histories, we had stories we passed down through generations in oral histories. You can read about history in a book, but you will remember the stories you experienced longer. We have developed many ways for people to experience stories. You can tell someone verbally not to drink and drive, but presenting a multi-sensory story about a drunk driver will have more impact. A story stays in your memory better than information and facts do. A life without stories is not a life worth living.

We have added more reality to our stories since the times of the Greeks and Shakespeare. They may have depicted actual people, but they were not normal people living regular lives. The storytellers represented kings, queens, and other powerful people as characters. They were often powerful people because historians wrote about their histories. They may have told stories of everyday people, but examples of these stories have only recently surfaced. The stories have gone from pure entertainment to a more poignant and realistic view of people's lives.

People who read, watch, or listen to a wide variety of stories are more empathetic than those who only watch the news or factual based programs. Stories connect us as people. It is hard to watch a story about a certain group of people and feel hatred toward them. A hateful person will only watch stories about people they do not hate. People may perceive stories differently, but the story will connect with more people who connect with the emotions of the story. Connecting with stories is the same as connecting with other people. People who do not enjoy stories do not enjoy people.

Stories about unfamiliar groups of people will give you a better understanding of their life. When you see the similarities and differences, you will develop an understanding of the culture and people in it. If the group is only a part of a bigger story, you may not get their genuine stories. They may only be a stereotype of the group from outsiders. Experiencing one person or a few people's stories is not a complete picture of them. The more stories you hear about them, the better you will understand them.

Stories can be about a single person or multiple people. The fewer people in the story, the better you can get to know each of the characters. I am a much bigger fan of intimate stories than epic ones. An epic story involves too many people to get to know individually. You can get an impression of a society from a different time or place, but you do not get to know them deeply. Personal stories allow us to understand the experiences that formed a person's life.

Some stories are compassionate toward the characters in them, and others are critical of them. Compassionate stories help us understand the people in the stories. They are realistic views of the life of a group of people told from members of the group or people who knew them. Critical stories provide us with a lesson about a group of people or person. They do not tell an authentic story. The storytellers use them to tell others how to live. They are morality tales meant to instruct others. We populate them with heroes and villains instead of authentic people. Compassionate stories represent reality, and critical stories represent the beliefs of their creators.

The popularity of a story depends on how you tell the story. A story told well will have a larger audience than one told poorly. We have valued excellent storytellers throughout history. They are experts on what makes a story interesting and entertaining. When you experience a story told well, you will want to hear other stories from the storyteller. Storytelling expresses emotional truths no other form of entertainment can express. Emotional songs, dances, or other forms of entertainment are emotional because they tell a story. Stories keep us connected to one another. People are not "other people" when you know their story.

We like simple things when we are kids like sports, superheroes, and simple comical stories. As we grow up, we like more complex things like science, learning, and complex stories. If you only like simple stories as an adult, you have not grown as a person. We may dig deeper into stories we thought were simple and find deeper meanings, but we are always growing more complex as people. When we focus more on the facts and details of a story than the story itself, we miss the point of the story. We can tell the same story with completely diffcrent details and it remains the same. We connect to stories just as we connect to other people. Thc story creates a relationship between the characters in them and us.

The characters in stories help us stay in touch with our own humanity. You can learn how to behave from them without having to know them as actual people. We can only learn so many lessons from our parents or mentors about how to behave with other people. Angry characters teach us as much as content ones. Characters present examples of what to do or not to do. We learn more from characters who grow than ones who do not change throughout a story. Even non-human characters can teach us about ourselves.

The Reality of Fiction

Fictional stories can present a greater emotional reality than a story based on actual people or historical events. They allow us to get to know characters through their actions. We do not know their history and have no preconceived conceptions of them. This is how we get to know the people we meet in our lives. We will relate to some people and not others. They are fictional, but they become actual people in our minds. Many fictional writers create back-stories for their characters the audience does not know about. They can base the characters on actual people in an authentic place or fictional creatures from a fictional world. Fictional stories allow the storytellers' skills to shine or their flaws to become apparent.

I liked fantasy stories as a kid because I did not like the reality of my life. Seeing genuine people struggling with life was not as enjoyable as seeing fantasy creatures dealing with their own struggles. I could accept the reality of their life and ignore my own struggles. The reality depicted in the stories was not the reality I lived in. Their world operated by different rules. The characters took for granted what the audience must discover for themselves. I liked these stories because they presented a world whose rules I understood. I did not have the skills to understand the rules of the world I lived in.

Fiction can help you accept reality. You can view a fictional reality from a distance. You are not living in a fictional world, but you can learn from it. Life can happen so fast that you do not have time to understand it. We must understand a fictional story to enjoy it. You can understand life in a fictional world which can help you understand your own life. A fictional character cannot hide being miserable from an audience who are experiencing their thoughts or private moments. When people are having tough moments, they can suppress their negative thoughts and put a smile on their face. Fiction allows us to accept the insecurities we all have and deal with them.

Inappropriate behavior from fictional characters is entertaining. They break the rules we know would have consequences in actual life. We only see the characters dealing with the consequences if it is integral to the story. We may see characters misjudging others for their behavior. In a fictional society that does not accept reality, they judge behavior with their collective beliefs. The fictional story allows the audience to view people's behaviors from the outside. If a child interrupts a business meeting, it is more natural behavior than the behavior of the members of the meeting. There is no logical reason for people to dress in business suits and discuss third quarter revenues. We can see this absurd behavior as illogical compared to the child's natural behavior in a fictional story.

Taking fiction seriously misses the point of fiction. Saying things are not realistic in a fictional work is to misunderstand the word "fiction." If a work has a few unbelievable elements, it is science fiction. If it has many unbelievable elements, it is a fantasy. The only rules authors cannot break in fiction are the rules established by them when they begin their stories. If they establish that Earth's gravity exists and people fly around, they have broken their own rules.

We created fiction to entertain with its emotional reality. Understanding fiction helps us understand reality.

Reality Accepting Exercise:

Think about a story from your past others would not believe because it was so unbelievable. You may even question whether it actually happened. What was it about the event that made it so unbelievable? Do you think the story has changed from the first time you told it? When you tell the story, do you exaggerate certain details to make it more exciting? If you were to make a scene in a movie about the event, what would you have to add or take away? Does a story have to be realistic to be entertaining?

Stories from your life are never an exact retelling of events as they happened. We think of ourselves as reliable witnesses and maybe we are, but the reality of any event does not make an interesting story. Stories entertain us. We do not tell stories to present the most accurate portrayal of reality. Some people can only state facts about events, but those facts do not make entertaining stories. Experiencing other people's stories helps relieve us of the realities of our lives. Seeing your life as a story will help keep you interested in your life.

Chapter 29
Solving Problems with Reality Acceptance

Reality Acceptance Problem Solving Method

The scientific method can solve any problem. Reality Acceptance uses the scientific method to show you how you can know what reality to accept. The following page is a comparison of the basics of the scientific method and concrete steps from Reality Acceptance you can use to solve problems in your life.

Scientific Method	Reality Acceptance Method
Ask a question	What is the reality of this situation?
Do background research	Ask questions and gather information from various sources.
Construct a hypothesis	Use the information to form a logical conclusion that considers the most factors about the situation.
Test with an experiment	Test your conclusions in the real world one by one to see what works, what only partially works, and what does not work.
Analyze data	Analyze the real-world tests for the results that satisfy the most factors involved in the situation.
Form conclusion and publish results	Talk to other people about your results and get their input. Change your conclusions if necessary and test the conclusions in the actual world again.

Solutions

All of life is a series of problems we need to solve. From the time we take our first step to dealing with the end of our life, problems present themselves for us to solve. The fewer problems you solve in life, the lower your ability to solve problems. We must accept the reality of any problem before we can begin thinking about how to solve it. Misunderstanding or ignoring part of a problem will lead to unresolved problems. We can use Reality Acceptance to find solutions to our problems.

Finding solutions does not mean those solutions work for everyone. We need to make compromises on problems involving larger groups of people. The solutions helping the most people will be the best solutions. Most societal problems stem from past solutions that only considered a few of the people involved in them. War is a solution that only solves problems for people in power. Most of the society will only find themselves with more problems, with no help from those in power. Our solutions must solve hard problems to help the most people.

Solutions ignoring major factors of a problem will not solve the problem. They may solve a portion of the problem, but not much more than doing nothing. We may need several solutions to solve complex problems. Societal problems are always complex. We may have individual problems stemming from the societal problems, but the societal problems are a major factor we cannot ignore. Solutions that examine the most factors of a problem will be better solutions.

Solving problems begins with examining basic realities and working your way to more complex ones. You start with basic problems when you are figuring out what is wrong with a computer. These are usually power or connection issues. The basics for a human are physical and mental health issues. These issues will manifest as behaviors based on biases, beliefs, and hidden agendas. When these issues spread throughout a group or society, they will expand into societal problems. We can solve these problems or prevent them with Reality Acceptance.

Complex problems require solutions from several sources and an acceptance of the combined solutions. We need to solve multiple problems together to solve complex problems. The more problems that interact with one another, the harder they are to solve individually. Problems do not present themselves one at a time, so you can solve one before you move on to the next. Prioritizing problems is necessary. The more we understand the reality of the problems, the better we can find solutions. Complex problems can appear like a jigsaw puzzle without a colorful picture. Reality is the picture you must understand before you can solve the puzzle.

Following is a list of problems and solutions using the Reality Acceptance Method. I present them to give you an idea of how Reality Acceptance can solve real-world problems. If you think of better solutions, I have done my job in this book.

How do I handle my negative emotions?

Negative emotions such as anger, sadness, and anxiety will only get worse if we ignore them. They will lead to negative behaviors that will degrade your health. Your negative emotions come from your experiences, traumas, and beliefs.

They are usually from a time in your life when you had less control. Admitting you have these negative emotions is the first step to fixing them. Examine recent times you have had negative emotions or behaviors. Did your behavior reflect the reality of the situation, or were they exaggerated because of your emotions? You cannot change the traumas of the past, but you can change your behavior in the present. Every experience is a chance to improve your reaction to these emotions and change the emotions you feel. If you have trouble examining your negative emotions, find someone who can help you with them.

What can I do about my physical health problems?

If you have existing physical problems, it may be too late to improve your physical health fully. Physical problems start from the basics. If you do not eat nutritious foods, drink plenty of water, and exercise daily, start now. Both your mental and physical health will improve. When you notice specific physical aches or pains, research ways to eliminate the pain and begin strengthening the muscles in that area. If you injure yourself doing a dangerous activity, stop doing that activity! I am sure you enjoy skiing while juggling knives, but it is not good for your health. Keeping yourself safe and physically active will prevent or improve most health problems. If you are in the "too late" category, see a doctor. They will be able to help.

What can I do about my mental health problems?

Mental health problems are more difficult than physical problems. Your mental health is usually only noticeable to others in your behavior. If you behave with extreme anger, sadness, or anxiety to normal situations, it is a sign of mental instability. If you are stressed, have sleeping problems, yell often, or bring drama with you everywhere you go, you have mental health problems. The reasons behind your unhealthy behaviors stem from emotional experiences from your past you have not dealt with.

The actual experiences are not as important as recognizing these emotional events are affecting your current emotional health and your behavior. You can use your behavior to recognize your emotional state. You can also use others' behaviors to recognize their emotional states. As you continue recognizing your emotions and dealing with them, you will have less unhealthy behaviors. Mental health is not a game you win, but a practice that improves over time. If your mental health problems are severe, see a mental health professional or someone who is mentally healthy.

How can I handle stress?

No feeling will harm your health as much as stress. An overwhelming amount of physician visits are stress related. It can cause anger, sadness, and anxiety, which can lead to more health problems. Much of stress is self-imposed. A major source of stress is feeling a lack of control in your life. Much of this lack of control happens at work, but it can happen anywhere. Money can be a factor in stress, but it is the lack of control of money that causes the stress. Many of the richest people are the most stressed.

Dealing with stress is a matter of understanding the emotions causing your stress. An emergency is inherently stressful. Keeping a situation from becoming stressful is a matter of not becoming overwhelmed and knowing your limitations. Do not handle too many issues at once. The human mind can only handle one problem at a time. The rest of what we do is automatic and does not require conscious thought. No situation requires a stressful response. We can handle all of life's situations without stress, but we must learn to deal with and remove our stressful habits.

Why do I always feel exhausted?

Exhaustion comes from overexerting yourself. Knowing your limits is key to avoiding exhaustion. There are physical and mental limits to what your body and brain can handle. Unless you are in an emergency, there is no reason to exhaust yourself. Most people are unaware when they are exhausted. They are doing what they have done in the past, but this time they get exhausted. The person's age, health level, amount of sleep deprivation, and several other factors can explain why this activity causes exhaustion.

People often overexert themselves if they see someone else doing an activity without getting exhausted. They ignore the stress on their body until it completely exhausts them. Exhaustion is your body's way of telling you to stop and rest. Heart attacks, headaches, strained muscles, and many other problems can come from ignoring your body's message. Take your exhaustion seriously and see a health professional if it is severe.

How can I avoid feeling so confused all the time?

Confusion is not understanding a situation. Most confusion is not understanding several things at once. When you find yourself confused, think about what you understand. Start with the basics of a situation and build what you know about it until you come to something you do not understand. You may find a single aspect of something is confusing you. Finding others who can help you understand things is important. There are some things you may never fully understand. Unless you depend on those things to live, you may never need to understand them. Quantum physics still confuses me, but I understand it enough to know my life is fine without fully understanding it.

How do I keep myself from feeling alone?

Feeling isolated, alone, or withdrawn is something every person has dealt with in their life. Most of the time, we feel it when we are not actually alone. We feel alone because we do not connect to other people. When people say they like to be alone, they have purposely disconnected themselves from other people. Connecting with other people makes us vulnerable. If you are never vulnerable with other people, you will never connect with them.

We do not connect with other people because others have mistreated us in the past. We isolate ourselves from others to protect ourselves. When you see people who remind you of those who mistreated you, you feel alone. Dealing with those feelings is a matter of understanding why they mistreated you. It had nothing to do with you. They were behaving as they did because of their own insecurities. When surrounded by people you do not know, it is an opportunity to get to know new people. Everyone feels as insecure as you do when you first meet them, but you will both be better off if you can connect as people.

How can I pay attention when I have difficulty concentrating?

Having difficulty concentrating can have several causes. It is important to understand why you are having difficulties. When are you finding it difficult to concentrate? Where do you have difficulties concentrating? Are there certain people you cannot concentrate around? If you can concentrate while in a situation, examine it to find out what is different. When you find barriers to your concentration, brainstorm solutions to eliminate those barriers. Get help from others to help you remove them. The more you pinpoint and deal with the barriers, the better you can concentrate. If you still cannot concentrate, you may need professional help.

How can I shake my addiction?

Addictions come in many forms. They can be as small as a donut addiction or as large as a cocaine addiction. All addictions stem from traumas you have not dealt with. Until you deal with the trauma that turned your habit into an addiction, you cannot deal with your addiction. Your addiction may relate to the trauma, or it may merely be a coping mechanism to deal with the trauma. Acknowledging and dealing with the trauma is a crucial step.

Admitting to yourself you have a problem is easier than admitting to others you have a problem. When you work up the courage to tell others, you will find they already know. They may not know about your specific addiction, but they know there is a problem. Most people will help you with your addiction. If someone is not willing to help, find someone who is. Making yourself accountable to others will make you accountable to yourself. Eliminating the habit completely is not as critical as acknowledging when your habit is the strongest. Replacing your unhealthy habits with healthy habits will help you deal with cravings.

Many addictions are not simple habits we can stop or avoid. Physical addictions require outside help. You must find people you trust to get the help you need. Most addictive substances have programs that can help you. Any resistance you feel toward the programs will prevent them from working. You must find a program that works for you. Whenever you have bad days, remember today is always better than yesterday. It may not feel like it, but getting back to yourself before your addiction took over your life always feels better.

How do I get help with my sleeping problems?

Most people have difficulty sleeping in their life. Understanding your sleep problems begins with examining how you sleep. What are you doing before you sleep? Do you have other difficulties like stress you are dealing with? Do you have a tough time relaxing throughout your day? Most of us do not have problems sleeping in the right circumstances. The key is finding the optimal circumstances for avoiding sleep problems.

The first thing to examine is your sleeping environment. If it is too loud, quiet, bright, dark, or any other form of distraction, you will not sleep well in it. If you sleep well in that same environment at other times, it is something else. Next, examine your routine around sleeping. Do you do different things on nights when your sleeping is worse? Experiment with your routine to see if a change works better. When you find things that work for you, make them part of your sleep routine.

How do I talk to people I disagree with?

Disagreeing with other people is part of life. Everyone's perceptions are different, so disagreements are inevitable. We usually know what topics are contentious to talk about with people we know. The best thing to do is avoid those topics. They will not change your mind and you will not change theirs. There are an endless number of topics people can talk about, so why focus on the few contentious ones?

Some people engage in conversations who only know you disagree with them. They want you to debate them so they can prove you wrong. These debates will only end up in more disagreements. The best policy is to decline the debate politely. You may suggest another topic you both agree on, but people looking for a debate are not usually looking for a conversation. If they bring things up around you to tempt you into a debate, you may need to remove yourself from them.

The most difficult contentious conversations are those with your supervisors or caregivers. They have power over you that other people do not. If they want you to agree with them, you must be diplomatic about your answers. You do not have to lie, but you also do not have to express all your thoughts to them. Not explicitly disagreeing with them is the best thing to do. Countering their opinions with facts will not help the situation. They think of their opinions as facts. You can debate the source of their facts, but that will not help either. You do not have to like or care about their opinions when you are no longer under their control.

How do I keep myself from procrastinating?

Procrastination happens when we force people to do things they do not want to do. We procrastinate doing chores and come up with excuses for not doing them. To prevent yourself from procrastinating, you need to understand what part of the chore you dislike. Is there a way you can do it you would like more? You can tell yourself you do not have to finish the chore all at once. Find parts of the chore you like to do more. Do those first. We concentrate on the boring parts of a chore to talk ourselves out of starting it.

Part of doing chores is planning how you will do them. This can be the part we dread the most. Breaking the chore into smaller actions can prevent you from becoming overwhelmed. Start with simple actions and build to more complex ones. If the chore is boring, entertain yourself while you work with something you find stimulating. You can listen to music, audiobooks, or other audio shows. You can also involve someone else to help you or just keep you company. Avoiding procrastination is about working your way through the chore in whatever way works best for you. You get the chore done, but your way.

How do I handle people with antisocial behavior?

Antisocial behavior can come from people who do not care about other people or themselves. They are antisocial because they believe society is against them. Their behavior shows inner turmoil. They do not ask themselves if they should do something, they only ask if they want to do it. You can help them if you can convince them you care about them as people. You also need to find out if they are aware of their behavior. Making assumptions about people is the quickest way to misunderstand them. Find out who they are and you will find out why they behave as they do.

Ironically, many people crave the negative attention they receive from society. Part of helping them is not giving them the attention they are craving. It may not make sense to you why they would crave negative attention, but it makes sense to them. If you punish them, you are proving to them that society does not care about them. Showing you care about them will show them it is their behavior that society discourages or misunderstands, not them. We all want to connect with other people, but some of us do not know how to do it. Show them you can overlook their inappropriate behavior and get to know them as people.

How do I prevent someone from discriminating against others?

Racism, sexism, class-discrimination, and other discriminatory practices stem from the societies we live in. Unless you are part of a movement to end these practices, there is little you can do to change collective thinking. Discrimination of any kind comes from a misunderstanding of a group of people or a person. We have all experienced discrimination in our lives. Whether you are conscious of it depends on how frequently the discrimination takes place. If you experience constant discrimination, you know you are in a discriminated group. The discrimination can seem like a normal part of our life, but it is not normal or acceptable.

Take notice when people are discriminating against other people. You may not know how to change the discrimination, but you can talk to those discriminated against. Let them know you noticed the discrimination and tell them you will help them if you can. Ignoring discrimination is ignoring other people. If your friends are discriminating against others, talk to them about it. Point out the behavior to them and help them see that their behavior is harmful to all.

How can I convince others to accept reality?

The best thing we can do for other people is talk to them. You need not explain the concepts of Reality Acceptance to them. You only need to talk to them about the concept of understanding reality. Find out how they determine if something is real. Tell them your thoughts, but do not present yourself as an authority on reality. It took me an entire book to explain Reality Acceptance. You will not convince them to accept reality in one conversation. Getting them to think about their understanding of reality is a good start. Find realities they accept and use those to talk about their understanding of reality.

Some people do not want to accept reality. They have spent their lives only accepting simple versions of reality they can understand. You can still engage them in a discussion of what makes them happy. Some people will never accept the reality of their health, but most people know what makes them happy. There are people who do not think happiness is worth pursuing. This is sad, but true. I would not give up on these people. Show them you care about them and be an example of what happiness looks like. If they eventually see the value of happiness, you can start discussing other realities.

Reality Accepting Exercise:

Think about how you solved a major problem in your life. Did you have help in solving the problem? Did you solve other problems in the same way? Was the solution more or less of a compromise than you were expecting? Did it give you confidence to solve other problems? Would you solve the same problem differently if it happened today? Did you find the challenge of solving the problem exciting, scary, annoying, or some other emotional feeling? Do you offer suggestions when you hear others trying to solve similar problems?

Everyone can solve problems in their lives. The quality of those solutions varies wildly. Thinking you have the best solution for any circumstance ignores most of the factors involved in any problem. Solving one problem involves solving other problems related to the fundamental problem. The best solution is never best for everyone. Everyone involved must make compromises. Minimizing the number of compromises for all involved is key to making the best solution.

Chapter 30
Conclusion

I began noticing more people who need this book when I was about halfway through writing it. It gave me the incentive I needed to finish it. They were not accepting the reality of their stressed out and miserable lives. I told people, "I talk about this in my book," and knew I could never encompass the concepts of Reality Acceptance in a single conversation. My inability to articulate my thoughts in a conversation was hampering my ability to make myself understood. This book was the accumulation of all the incomplete conversations I have had with many different people.

I hope this book will be the beginning of spreading Reality Acceptance to anyone who wants to be happier and healthier. It is a simple concept with many possibilities for changing the world. No one is miserable or unhealthy because they want to be. We are that way because we believe it is our reality. We do not have separate realities. Reality is something we must consciously attempt to understand. It is a goal that luckily never ends. People who think they have all the answers are accepting simple and boring answers. Understanding reality is the most exciting thing we can pursue in our lives.

Reality Acceptance can improve every aspect of our lives. I hope we can someday include it in psychology, education, public policies, and anywhere people are trying to improve their lives. Most of this book concerned improving our lives individually, but there is no reason we cannot improve all societies everywhere. Improving your own life is just the beginning of your journey. I want you to continue collecting stories from as many diverse voices as you can. Our collective stories of discovery make life exciting.

We are all limited by time. I am no exception. My journey will only end when my brain stops being able to accept new realities. This book is the start of an unending conversation. People will disagree with concepts in this book, but it will hopefully begin more conversations. I did not tell you about reality; I told you how to understand reality. Science has advanced our understanding of reality more than any one person. I attempted to connect many modern scientific and social concepts to show the importance of understanding reality and valuing time. We all must value our own time just as much as we value the time of others.

I have only focused on realities that help us become happier and healthier. In the grand scope of understanding reality, they only represent a minor part. They are, however, important concepts many people do not think about. Helping people think about these concepts is the best way I can express how I care about them. These are not just words I believe to be true; they are ideas I know are true. I am living a life without hate. There are moments of anger and sadness, but they do not last. I experience negative emotions from other people and they affect me negatively. Striving to eliminate these negative emotions from as many people as we can is the most we can hope for.

You can continue finding out about current versions of Reality Acceptance at the Reality Acceptance website (**www.RealityAcceptance.com**). The website is a placeholder for present and future happenings. There are always new realities to accept. Return to the website whenever you want to get the latest information. There are many things I could not present in this book. The Internet is much more interactive than a book. There are resources, articles, and other helpful information to continue learning about Reality Acceptance. Please contact me at the website to talk about your thoughts about the book or your thoughts on reality. Reality!

Reality Accepting Exercise:

This last exercise is to continue your reality accepting journey beyond this book. I include Additional Resources at the end of the book. Look for reality accepting resources at the RealityAcceptance.com website and start noticing other reality accepting resources in your daily life. I am always looking for people to join me to expand Reality Acceptance to help more people accept reality and become their happiest and healthiest selves.

Acknowledgements

There are many people and groups I would like to acknowledge who helped me author this book. Here is an incomplete list of them.

Thank you to my wife and her family, who I feel are just as much my family as hers.

I thank my parents, who always allowed me to question everything they told me.

Thank you to all the co-workers I have had who, whether they knew it, put up with my hours of writing.

I thank all the friends who tolerated my conversations about accepting reality.

I thank all the reality accepting experts who taught me about the realities they have accepted.

I thank all the reality deniers in my life who showed me many examples of how not to live.

I thank all the cats my wife and I helped to raise for adding more happiness to my life.

Additional Resources

You can find out more about Reality Acceptance website at:

www.realityacceptance.com

There are many resources that helped me create this book. These resources include reality accepting experts, books, movies/videos, podcasts, series, and websites. I included them on the Reality Acceptance website at:

www.realityacceptance.com/category

You can also join my Facebook page at:

www.facebook.com/RealityAcceptancePage

You can find more information about the book and sign up for the Reality Acceptance Newsletter at:

www.realityacceptance.com/ra-book

About the Author

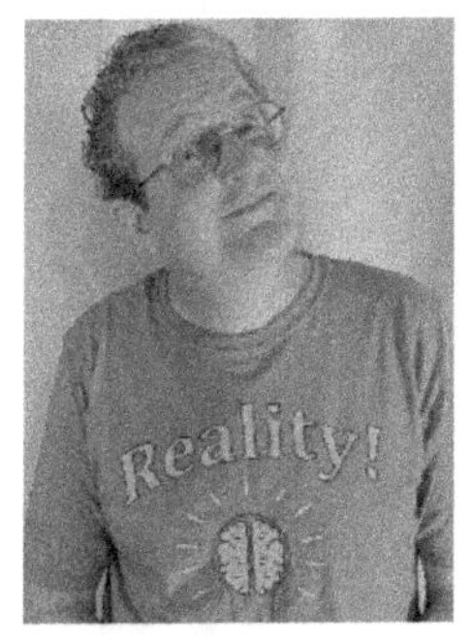

Brian Kirwan is a writer, composer, artist, filmmaker, and animator. He was born and raised in a small town in Southern California. As a child, he accepted realities most people ignored or denied. Growing up in a reality denying world proved difficult. Shyness, undiagnosed autism, and anxiety did not help. He was reaching the age of 50 when he realized he was tired of having to ignore the reality denial of other people and began his reality accepting journey. He noticed people who denied realities in their lives were not happy or healthy. The concept of Reality Acceptance came out of his desire to help others accept realities for themselves to improve their lives as he had done. It started as a website (**www.RealityAcceptance.com**) and developed into this book.